AF251700

Fight The Misery Conspiracy

Fight The Misery Conspiracy
Reclaiming Your Right to Be Happy

Dharmashanti

To Eileen,
My "happily ever after"

Acknowledgments

This is where I thank all of the people who have inspired me and who have helped me actually write this book and get it into your hot, little hands. Unless you actually know me, you might as well skip ahead to the introduction. No, really. Go on! Okay, now you're starting to creep me out. I'm getting a serious Kathy Bates "I'm your greatest fan" vibe, so put that sledgehammer down and move on. What was the name of that movie she was in? Oh yeah! *Misery!*

Now that all of my rabid fans have moved on to the more meaty portions of the book, there are a few people I'd like to thank. Let's see if you're one of them

First of all, I want to thank my mentor, Kaay Grosso. Your wisdom, guidance, creativity and generosity have helped me to overcome my personal demons and have shown me how to mentor others.

I want to thank my writing buddy/storyteller extraordinaire Audrey Lee who has helped me learn to speak Dharmish and pushed me to make my work the very best it can be.

I want to thank all of the women of the Garden Club and Emergence women's circles, whose diverse perspectives and experience have given me new ways to see the world.

I also want to thank Gen-la Kelsang Gyatso, Marianne Williamson, Richard Bach, His Holiness the Dalai Lama, Neale

Donald Walsch, my parents, my in-laws, my ex-husband, Ray, and my cats Panda (ngow!), Gizmo (meow!), and Lexie (peep!). You all have contributed to my life in so many special ways.

Most of all, I want to thank my wife, Eileen. You were the best unexpected blessing of my life. I couldn't possibly express in words how profoundly you have touched my heart. I wish everyone could find the Love we share.

Blessings and thanks to you all!

—Dharmashanti

Contents

Introduction

Your body aches from activities only half-remembered, while your mind still feels a bit gloopy. This can only mean one thing: it's Monday morning. Your supervisor raises an eyebrow as you pass her office, letting *you* know that *she* knows that you're 10 minutes late. "Screw her!" you say to yourself.

As you wait for the coffee maker to brew a fresh pot (because some time-pressed narcissist took the last cup and didn't start a new one), you run into your co-worker, Marcy. She mumbles an acknowledgment.

"Okay for a Monday," you reply, just guessing she asked how you were.

Yeah, you're doing "okay," considering it's Monday. You're at work. Money's tight. Your ex is suing you for custody of your chihuahua...again. Your girlfriend or boyfriend (or both) is a nag. Your Mercedes Benz is in the shop...again. Your pants are too tight. Your boss has denied your request for a raise...again. Aliens have implanted a chip in your brain ...again. Does any of this sound familiar? Okay, except for the Mercedes.

You *think* that all of these problems in your life are the reasons why you're not Happy. And why not? You've been raised in a train-wreck society, populated by others who think the same way. They are stupid, inconsiderate and will do anything to bring you down. Unless you have the combined temperament of Mother

Theresa and the Dalai Lama, this place gets to you. How can anybody be Happy with so much crap going on?

Well, that is, in fact, a very interesting question. How can you be Happy when life is so full of disappointment and injustice? The thing that makes this question so interesting is that it contains within it an assumption that is at the root of your unhappiness. This is the threshold of the Misery Conspiracy.

Mind you, there's nothing wrong with blaming your misery on your circumstances. Nothing wrong with it at all, unless, of course, you would rather be *Happy*. But who wants that? This is *your* misery! You own it and no one can take it away from you, not even God. Doesn't the U.S. Constitution guarantee you the right to life, liberty and the pursuit of misery?

What's that? You *want* to be Happy? Really? Well, in that case you should be warned that being Happy and Joyful and Peaceful is subversive. It's contrary to the status quo. Happiness isn't normal. People will think you're weird or stoned or just plain crazy. They may even try to take advantage of your generosity and compassion. Are you sure you can take that kind of pressure? Can you handle the Truth?

Okay, maybe you can. But be aware that Happiness, *real* Happiness, isn't cheap. It's going to cost you a lot to attain True Joy and Peace. You'll have to give up your resentments, hatred, self-pity, prejudices, projections and delusions about everything! You may even have to forgive people you don't like. We're talking serious sacrifice here; not to mention the extensive time and effort involved. Surely it's not worth all that just to find Joy and Serenity and, Heaven forbid, Love. After all, if it was really worth it, wouldn't everybody already be doing it?

Hmmm. You're still reading, so maybe you do have what it takes. Maybe. So let's start with a simple, yet subversive truth. Ready? Here it is.

You don't need a reason to be happy.

Unbelievable, isn't it? It doesn't matter how unfair life is or how many injustices you have to endure. It doesn't matter what your stepfather did to you or how little money you have or what you look like. You can be Happy in spite of it all.

What no one has told you (or maybe they did and you didn't believe them) is that your Happiness, Joy and Serenity are a choice you make every moment of the day. If that seems oversimplified, it's because you have been brainwashed to think so. That's the Misery Conspiracy at work! It's designed to keep you in the dark and to keep you miserable.

So what's all this talk about conspiracy? Sounds kinda paranoid, doesn't it? But as the saying goes, "Just because you're paranoid, doesn't mean someone's not out to get you!" A conspiracy is a collective agreement to deceive or to conceal the truth about something. And folks, call me paranoid or call me a heretic, but there is a worldwide conspiracy to keep you miserable.

What is the Misery Conspiracy? It's a lie – the biggest lie. It is the granddaddy of all urban legends! If an ego is the personification of our selfish thoughts, then the Misery Conspiracy is the negative synergy created from a world run by egos. It is the deadly undertow that pulls our unsuspecting spirits into the murky depths of despair. Glub, glub, glub.

In less abstract terms, the Misery Conspiracy is a worldwide belief system, based on lovelessness, fear and deception. This flawed belief system has infiltrated nearly every aspect of human life. It's in our governments. It's in our businesses and schools. It's even in our places of worship. Surprise! It has so thoroughly penetrated our culture that we usually rarely notice it. We have this gnawing feeling that something is wrong, but we can't put our finger on the real issue.

The Misery Conspiracy sends you looking for Love and Happiness and Serenity in all of the places they can't be found. It distracts you from your own power by sending you on wild goose chases in hopes of acquiring that "next thing" or that "one person" you hope will make you Happy, but never does. How many of us have been there? Yeah, that's what I thought. We all have. Imagine that!

Then the Misery Conspiracy consoles us with, "That's okay. The *next* thing will make you Happy. Mr. or Ms. Right is out there! Keep looking in bars, at raves, and on the internet, because you can't be Happy until you find them and make them fall in love with you." Rather than learn our lesson, we go panting off like the good little puppies we are, chasing after the stick that never got thrown. Arff!

Perhaps you're wondering who's behind the Misery Conspiracy? Who is this evil Axis of Ego, bent on denying us our Joy? Good question! Is it the politicians? Yes! Is it the corporations and the lobbyists? Absolutely! Is it the teachers and the preachers? You better believe it. And here's the clincher! Brace yourself! You, too, are a conspirator and so am I. We all are responsible for the Misery Conspiracy. We bought into it as kids and have been keeping the blind faith ever since.

Evidence of this conspiracy is everywhere. (Imagine that! A conspiracy theory with actual evidence!) Watch CNN for an hour and count how many negative stories there are. Add to that the number of commercials that tell you that you can't be Happy unless you buy their product or service. From your current total, subtract the number of really heinous-looking newscasters or female anchors over the age of 40 (hint: ZERO). You might want to get a calculator.

Look at the insane popularity of "reality television" and crime dramas. Now ask yourself why we as a society, and more importantly why YOU as an individual, are so addicted to other people's drama and misery. Why is it so fascinating? It's the Misery Conspiracy!

The conspiracy is so pervasive that we don't notice it most of the time, in the same way that we are rarely conscious of the pull of gravity or the rotation of the earth or the way our waistlines steadily expand (or maybe that's just me). We're unaware of this social and spiritual addiction to the negative.

We are absolutely convinced we can't be Happy until something in our lives changes (new job, new lover, new baby, new car, more money, less fat, more hair in some places, less hair in other places, etc.). Either we believe we don't have the right to be Happy, or we doubt our ability to be Happy — at least right now.

We're like Neo caught up in the Matrix, with no clue that we've been living a nightmare of delusions. But unlike the Matrix, our dream world was self-created and reality isn't a dark, post-apocalyptic world. True Reality (yes, it seems redundant, but I'm trying to explain something, so pay attention!) is much brighter and the Real You is a Divine Presence that extends throughout the Universe. You are an extension of the Divine Consciousness of Unconditional Love, frequently referred to as God.

I'm losing you, aren't I? Talking about God is one thing, but then I had to go all New Age/New Thought on you, didn't I? Talk like "the world isn't real" is a bit much for most people. It sounds like some crazy conspiracy theory, right? Maybe you're thinking that I've watched *What the Bleep Do We Know* a dozen times too many. I admit it does sound pretty ridiculous.

What I have discovered, however, is that our perception of reality has been distorted. We've been raised to think that in order for us to have more, someone else must have less. According to the thinking of the Misery Conspiracy, the world is divided into predators and prey. We've been told that competition is better than cooperation and that the best defense is a good offense. But have these fearful, loveless, selfish philosophies given us a lasting sense of Joy and Peace? Not really! They've made us miserable.

Who started the Misery Conspiracy? Who knows! It really doesn't matter who started it. It only matters that we not perpetuate it. As prevalent as the lies of the Misery Conspiracy might be, we are not obligated to maintain them. We can fight the Misery Conspiracy and reclaim our right to Happiness! It's time to consider a different philosophy, and to open ourselves to a more enlightened perception of reality.

This enlightened viewpoint isn't new. It has been around for millennia. The consensus of history's most enlightened minds is that our essential nature is one of Unconditional Love. They have agreed, as well, that by connecting with the Consciousness of Love, we reach a state of kickass Bliss. Buddha taught this. So did Jesus, Rumi, the Bhagavad-Gita, Gandhi, Thoreau, Emerson, Mother Theresa, and the Dalai Lama. These and others are the voices of the Spiritual Revolution!

Power to the people! Fight the Conspiracy! Down with the ego! Off with its head! Grab the pitchforks and torches! Drag out the guillotine!

All right, maybe it's not that kind of revolution. In fact, that is the kind of mob mentality that we're looking to overcome, right? It's our own loveless thinking that is the problem — that whole "us versus them" insanity that we see throughout society. But our problem isn't with *them*. Our problem is who we think *they* are.

As with any revolution, we must arm ourselves with the proper tools. It does no good to shout for regime change and then bust through the gates unarmed. No, not with pitchforks or torches or even rolled up copies of the *Washington Post*. Not with clever clichés or insulting rhetoric or three-syllable talking points (like "Stay the Course", "Cut and Run" or "Kiss my Ass"). Our tools are much more powerful than that, and you don't have to be a genius to use them. Good thing, too, or I'd be in serious trouble!

Because our struggle for Peace is an *internal* one, the place where we have to do the most work is in our very own minds. We must use tools such as gratitude, meditation, prayer, and mindfulness, and learn to use them so well that they replace blaming, judgment and guilt as our weapons of choice. That is the purpose of this book: to teach you how to change your thinking and help you create a life that is powerful and joyous.

Let me conclude this introduction with a few clarifications. You will notice that I make references to the One Self here and there. The One Self is the place/state of consciousness where we are all connected. It is God and me and you and that jerk down the street that plays his stereo too loud. It's the Collective Consciousness of Unconditional Love. The One Self is that voice in your mind calling you to forgive, to let go of resentments, and to learn to love unconditionally. It is your True Self and your Spiritual Source.

Granted, chances are good that your concept of a Higher Power (another name for the One Self) differs from mine. You may call it Goddess, Allah or Jehovah. You might see it as our Buddha Nature or Krishna Consciousness or Christ Mind. Not a problem! If you believe in a Divine Presence, call it whatever feels right to you, and feel free to mentally substitute that name any time I refer to the One Self, God or our Spiritual Source.

You may not believe in any Divine Supreme Being at all. Again, not a problem. If you identify as agnostic or atheistic, just imagine the most enlightened, loving version of yourself, what some call your Highest Self. If you can't do any of the above, well, it's time to open that closed mind of yours to new possibilities. After all, if you had all the answers, would you be reading this book? Didn't think so.

However you conceive of the One Self (or God or Goddess or Buddha Nature or the Universe or the Great Green Arkleseizure), what really matters is re-connecting to it in a deeply emotional and spiritual way. Doing so changes the nature of our thinking at the most fundamental levels, which in turn changes the nature of our actions, ultimately transforming the Universe we see ourselves in.

As we consciously re-connect to the One Self, we begin to experience Joy, Peace and Love in ways we never imagined. It's the spiritual equivalent of finally getting hooked up with running water. It changes everything, including those scary midnight trips to the outhouse. Woo hoo!

Be warned, however! By countering the Misery Conspiracy's machinations, by pointing out the lies that we have always been told, you will encounter strong resistance, both internally and externally. By realizing your own Joy, you remind people how miserable they are. They may wonder what gives *you* the right to be so freakin' Happy. They may even attempt to drag you back down into the muck with them. Don't let this discourage you. Crazy people do crazy things, but you will learn that none of it has any permanent effect on you.

You will also have a tendency, especially at first, to fall back into old patterns. I still do in times of great stress or when I'm really tired. The Conspiracy doesn't go down quietly and will do everything it can to preserve its existence. In fact, just by reading this introduction, I suspect that the Conspirators of Misery have already written your name down. They may be tapping your phone.

These negative thought patterns will wait until things get a little out of hand, and will then begin playing those old tapes. Again, don't get discouraged. This is a spiritual *practice*! So just keep practicing! Perfection comes later, *much* later!!!

Another point of clarification is the capitalization of words like Love, Serenity, and Peace. I do this to emphasize the more divine, spiritual connotation of these words, as opposed to the cheaper, more casual, "Love ya! Mean it!" versions promoted by the Misery Conspiracy.

I understand that the word "Happy" means different things to different people. For some it's a temporary experience of pleasure, while for others it's simply an emotion. For the purposes of this book, however, I'm using it as a catch-all for the profound experiences of Joy, Serenity, Bliss, Peace, Unconditional Love, etc. These are all different expressions or forms of the same basic experience of the One Self. For simplicity purposes, I call it Happiness. Don't let the label confuse you. Just focus on the overall concept.

Finally, the stories and anecdotes that I share in the book are true. I am grateful for those whose lives have bumped into mine over the years, and who have provided great fodder for my book. In most cases, names have been changed to protect the anonymity of those mentioned. It's the least I could do (to make sure I have more juicy stories for my next book).

If you are tired of being miserable, if your bartender has put his kids through college on your bar tab, or if you have the suicide hotline on speed dial (been there, done that, got the stomach pumped!), it's time to recognize that you have been duped by the Misery Conspiracy! It's time to gather with like-minded people and recognize the truth. Joy, Serenity and Unconditional Love are yours for the taking. You need only be willing to see beyond the limits of your present thinking to a new way of being.

Fight The Misery Conspiracy is my gift to you (okay, not exactly a gift, you paid for it), with hopes and prayers that you will find at least one suggestion or concept that will help you discover Happiness for yourself. Take what you like and leave the rest. But keep the door open for some ideas to bounce around your noggin before you discard them. I have found that some wisdom has to soak into our minds slowly before we can really make sense of it.

May you find much Peace, Love, Joy and Serenity soon! ¡Viva la revolución!

Namaste,
Dharmashanti

Section One:
The Dirty Secrets of the Conspiracy

Chapter 1:
The Conspiracy of Misery

Contrary to what you might be thinking right now, I haven't always been a Happy, Peaceful person. In fact, I'm still not one of those folks who never gets upset, who is always full of that annoying, bubbly, "HAPPY, HAPPY, HAPPY" energy. Those people scare me! The truth is that for most of my life, I was a moderately depressed, occasionally suicidal, and often codependent little drunk girl with borderline personality disorder and dissociative tendencies.

I was nearly thirty before my life finally started to come together. By that time, I had been married twice, was spending a few nights a week getting trashed at a local lesbian bar, and had no hope for the future. I was an unwitting, yet devout follower of the Misery Conspiracy. That's when I hit bottom.

On the morning of July 8, 1996, I found myself in the emergency room, trying to rub enough neurons together to gain some insight into how I had ended up there. With my lips stained black from the charcoal milkshake and my skin pale from having my stomach pumped, I looked very Goth. All I was missing was an eyebrow piercing, a skull tattoo and a black T-shirt and I could have blended in with the skaters at the mall.

The ER staff at Phoenix Baptist Hospital had spent the past few hours counteracting the overdose of aspirin and whiskey I had consumed the night before. In addition to forcing me to drink the charcoal and jabbing my wrist with a syringe every thirty minutes to check blood gases, they also forced me to explain why I attempted suicide. I felt like I was being tortured into confessing my darkest secrets.

"What could be so bad," they asked me, "that you would want to take your life?" It was a legitimate question, but one for which I had no reasonable answer. Explaining desperate acts of insanity to a perfectly rational person is futile, at best. There simply is no common point of reference, or of reality, for that matter.

The fact is, I intentionally swallowed nearly three dozen aspirin and chased it with a half-bottle of Irish whiskey. Crazy? Naturally! But it was the only way I knew to stanch the overwhelming emotional pain that I had spent a lifetime fighting. Sane people may find using titanic doses of aspirin an odd way to deal with *emotional* pain, but it made perfect sense to me at the time. Such are the ways of the rationally impaired.

All of us have faced major traumas if we've been around long enough. Some of us have dealt with debilitating physical conditions or illnesses. Others have been sexually molested or physically abused. Maybe you suffered the loss of a loved one at an early age or lived through a major financial loss. Or worst of all, you may have been forced to read *Finnegan's Wake* in high school lit (sorry, Mr. Joyce, but someone had to say it).

Sooner or later, everyone encounters that heartbreak of the soul — that moment in life when our world blows us apart with all the gentleness and compassion of an I.E.D. In this world of cruelty, apathy and poverty, it is inevitable. And yet, within the depths of our minds, there is a knowing, a hazy memory that whispers, "This isn't where you belong. You were not meant to suffer. This struggle against the demands of an insane world is not what life is about." Admit it. You've heard this voice, too.

If a loving God really is the Creator of the Universe, then something has gone terribly wrong. This chaotic, predator/prey existence must have been made by someone else. Check the label. Maybe it was made in some Saipan sweatshop by miserable people living in horrendous conditions. That would explain a lot.

If God is the Supreme Being of Love, why would She/He create such a loveless world? Shouldn't we be experiencing the profound Bliss of Oneness with our Source right about now? Shouldn't we be experiencing Peace, Serenity, and Joy? Shouldn't the television shows be at least a little better than the ones we have?

If God had indeed created the world we see, we *would* be at Peace. But a loving God does not create a kingdom built on lovelessness. God created Paradise, and in case you hadn't noticed, this isn't it. Aldous Huxley once wrote, "Maybe this world is another planet's hell." I believe he may have been on to something.

There is a conspiracy afoot to deny us Peace, what *A Course in Miracles* calls our "natural inheritance." Like the Prodigal Son, we have wandered from our True Home and have been brainwashed to think that this kill-or-be-killed carnival is where we belong. We have been told, often in not so subtle ways, that we have somehow forfeited our right to sit at God's table, and instead must beg for any scraps that come our way. We have awakened in this strange existence, not knowing who, what, or where we are.

Now I realize that such a conspiracy may seem a little far-fetched. The idea of an organized effort that has transformed us into the miserable folks we are is a bit too much for most people to swallow. But have you ever had a dream that seemed real while you were dreaming it? Of course you have! Have you ever had a nightmare that left you gasping and shaky, even after you woke up? Thought so!

So if your night dreams seem real while you are in them, isn't it possible that what you think of as reality is actually just another dream? What if there really is a conspiracy to keep you in this miserable dream, discouraging you from questioning its reality and blocking you from the realization of your Divine Nature?

So now we must ask who organized this Conspiracy of Misery? Who would commit such an atrocity against us, the Divine Children of the Universe? Who has both the will and the ability to deny us what God would not? The short answer is that it was you! And it was me! It was each and every one of us.

Okay, so we didn't start it, but we *have* perpetuated it. We have ignored the evidence of a world gone mad and just played along, not realizing the consequences to our state of mind. We have been so snowed by these diabolical machinations that the Truth now seems to be fantasy. We have been told repeatedly by parents, teachers, peers, bosses, and the teller at the bank (who really has it in for you) that we can't be Happy now, that there is always some condition that we must meet or some item that we must possess in order to be at Peace.

Yet, even when we finally get whatever it was that we so *desperately* needed to be Happy, we find that there is *some other reason* to be upset. There is always some caveat of the ego, the fine print in our contract with the devil that denies us what is ours. We are both Faustus and Lucifer, going head-to-head with ourselves.

How pervasive is this Conspiracy? Judge for yourself. Below I have listed many of the lies that the Misery Conspiracy tells us. When you hear someone passing these off as truth, much less Divine Truth, you can be assured that they are (consciously or not) part of the Conspiracy. So don't believe them!

These lies include:

- You are not good enough, smart enough, thin enough, beautiful enough, rich enough, or righteous enough.
- You are your body/job/religion/possessions.
- In order for you to gain, someone else must lose.
- You are not Divine.
- You are guilty.
- God hates you for your mistakes.
- God needs you to fear and worship Him.
- God loves [men, whites, Christians, Catholics, Muslims, Republicans, etc.] more than He loves other people.
- God has a gender (and it's probably male).
- God has a list of unacceptable behaviors.
- God has an ego, and is thus offended by our mistakes or defiance.
- God sends people to Hell.
- You only have one life/incarnation to get it right or be damned to Hell for eternity.
- God wants to punish you.

- God vents His wrath through natural disasters and acts of terrorism.
- There is only one way to God/Heaven/Enlightenment.
- There is only one True Scripture, and it is the inerrant Word of God.
- Anger, judgment and/or violence in the name of God are righteous and justified.
- Men are holier than women.
- Women are holier than men.
- The end justifies the means.
- Might equals right.
- Violence can get you what you want.
- Someone or something outside of you can make you Happy.
- Judgment, unforgiveness, resentments, and worry can produce satisfying results.
- Fear can be a good thing.
- Love is weak or naïve.
- There are legitimate reasons not to Love someone.
- You need a reason to be Happy.
- You can't be Happy on a Monday.
- Work can't be enjoyable.
- Wealth and professional success are signs of either righteousness or corruption.
- You can control what other people do or think.

These beliefs and others like them have been used by individuals, governments, and religious organizations to deny you what is rightfully yours: Peace, Joy and Love. And if you have incorporated any of them into your own worldview, you are denying yourself and others the same thing. You have become a part of the Conspiracy, and you probably didn't even know it. Surprise!

But my friend, there is a revolution underway to overthrow this empire of the ego. Even while our insane personalities perpetuate this Conspiracy of Misery, there are those of us who are working to subvert its illusionary authority. We have heard that other voice; the one that speaks not of our guilt, but of our innocence. We are the Spiritual Underground, and we are taking over.

For too long we have plowed hip deep through the misery of our separated, guilt-ridden, and vulnerable self-concept. We have catered to its whims, believed its judgments and suffered its vengeance. It is now time to take our bearings, find a better tour guide, and work our way back home to the Paradise Café in downtown Heaven (the Café Dharmas are divine!). We no longer have to listen to the rants and shrieks of the ego. This other, gentler voice, which I call the One Self, will show us the way home.

From the perspective of the Misery Conspiracy, listening to the voice of the One Self is dangerous. And no wonder! After years of negative thinking, opening ourselves up to a more positive approach can seem scary. We've become so entrenched in our insane thought patterns that anything different seems chaotic and unsure.

We might hate our prison of misery, but to venture outside into the sunshine and soft grass of our Divine Nature frightens us. We're waiting for the other shoe to drop. We're convinced that at any moment the ground is going to open up and Hades is going to sweep us up in his black chariot and drag us down into the darkness. And then there *will* be Hell to pay!

If our internal demons weren't enough, there is a tendency in some religious institutions to discourage people from listening to what the One Self is telling them. Such institutions don't want people making spiritual decisions on their own. It's too risky. There is fear that the Voice of Love in the individual's mind might be contrary to the institution's doctrine of fear and guilt, and it almost invariably is. To trust and follow the One Self is an abomination to the mindset of the Misery Conspiracy.

Other religious groups discourage dissent by refusing to discuss how certain "holy" texts came to be in their current form. They prefer to perpetuate the myth that God just faxed it down from Heaven, complete with annotations and concordance. To challenge such a notion is to be labeled a heretic, a blasphemer and a liar. Such are the names the Misery Conspiracy has for those who speak the Truth.

I'm not saying that such religious scriptures are wrong or bad. In fact, most contain a lot of spiritual wisdom. But it is important to consider not only their compliance with current religious beliefs, but also their historical context. No original copies exist of the teachings of the Buddha or of the Bible or the Talmud or the Qur'an. The best that we have are copies of copies of copies of copies...well, you get the idea.

Comparing different copies of the same scriptures have revealed changes and errors. Bart Ehrman, a Biblical scholar, has reported that there are more variations in the earliest manuscripts of the Bible than there are words in the New Testament. That's a lot of variation. This is hardly surprising since the written form of many ancient languages didn't include things like vowels (Hebrew) or spaces or punctuation (Greek). There are also words, cultural contexts, and subtle connotations that are lost when presented in new languages and new cultures.

My point is, despite the fact that much wisdom can be gain from studying these texts, blindly accepting any religious scripture or doctrine as Absolute Truth without question sets us up for disaster. Any belief that doesn't hold up to honest scrutiny is probably best left on the side of the road on your Spiritual Journey.

It is up to us to resist the Conspiracy, to make a conscious choice to listen to that other voice, the One Self that tells us that we *are* worth loving. Doing so sets in motion a chain of events that changes not only our outlook on life, but the very nature of the Universe itself. It sounds very pie-in-the-sky, I know. But give it a try. It works.

When I walked around thinking I was worthless, I had few friends and no romantic relationships. Nobody wanted to be around me. *I* didn't even want to be around me. No wonder I was depressed and suicidal!

Yet when I became willing to listen to the Voice of Love and was willing to believe that I was worth loving, that I was awesome just as I was, the difference was startling. Opportunities opened up.

Friends appeared in droves. And suddenly the love of my life (i.e. my spouse) showed up unannounced. It's like I'd flipped a switch from "Loser" to "Worth Checking Out!" And all I did was listen to Love rather than lovelessness.

When the Misery Conspiracy says we are separate, guilty and vulnerable, the One Self is there to remind us that we are connected, innocent, and safe. All we have to do to hear its voice is to be willing to hear it. We need to be willing to let go of all of our loveless thoughts about ourselves, God, and each other. When we do this, all of our fears will vanish like a morning fog burned away by the summer sun. We awaken to our True Nature, our Christ Consciousness, and find ourselves once again One with our Source. This is how the Misery Conspiracy is overthrown and Truth re-established.

Chapter 2:
The Game of Distraction

Now that you've become somewhat acquainted with the Misery Conspiracy, it's time to get a glimpse of how this nasty little belief system works to keep you from your Joy. One way it does this is through the game called "Distraction," This is a clever game not unlike Chutes and Ladders, complete with tricks to lift you (albeit artificially) to great heights of temporary ecstasy, followed by sudden plunges into despair.

The Conspiracy's function in this is to keep you preoccupied with everything except what can *really* make you Happy. In this way, you stay miserable. By blindly playing this game, you are less likely to recognize the flawed logic that the Conspiracy feeds us every day through our own insane thinking. Sounds like a fun game, huh?

When I began working on this book, I had a wide range of thoughts and feelings about how it would turn out and what kind of reception it would get by critics and the public.

Will I sell lots of books? Will I get halfway through and quit? Will I travel around the country on a speaking tour, doing interviews on TV and radio talk shows? Will I quit my job prematurely when my book takes off, but then have to beg for it back when it suddenly tanks? Will I finally be able to buy that cabin in the mountains? Will I be able to call up all the people from high school who thought I was nothing and say, "Hey, dude! Look at me now!"? I have issues, I know.

I have worked on a number of major, long-term projects and actually managed to complete a few of them, including this one, obviously. With each project, my mind always goes on wild jags about how wonderful or how terrible the final outcome of the project will be. One minute I'm sure it's going to be my rising star and the next I'm already chucking it on top of my huge pile of failed efforts. I'm charmingly psychotic that way.

This is an experience common to a lot of people. Oh, you, too? What a surprise! In spite of the distractions, most of us manage to stay reasonably functional as we trudge toward our goal. It is, however, important to understand what's really going on so that we can overcome the challenges that these projects offer and not create any unnecessary problems.

In many ways, our minds are like people learning how to water ski (only without the skis, a speedboat or the need to get wet). Starting out, we are rather undisciplined and have little experience using the skills we need to stay upright. When I first learned to water ski (don't even try to get me on a pair of snow skis!), I took turns falling in every possible direction. First I'd lean too far forward. Splash! Next I'd lean too far backwards! Whoosh! I'd fall left. I'd fall right. I'd even manage to catch the skis in just the right position to launch me about ten feet into the air; a stunt I thankfully never repeated.

My point is that our minds do the same thing all the time. We rarely notice it on the little stuff, but when something important comes up, we become the emotional equivalent of a first-time skier. *Is she gonna call? Is he not gonna call? Did I do well in that job interview? Will I find a buyer for my house? Will my unborn child get into that exclusive daycare, so that it can get in that exclusive elementary school, so that it can then get into that exclusive high school, and then on to be Valedictorian of his class at the Ivy League College?* Our thoughts are flopping all over the place and not accomplishing anything productive. Consciously, we know this, yet we can't help worrying and we can't stop thinking about it.

It's not our fault, really. This is part of the Misery Conspiracy's "Game of Distraction." We have been trained from conception to play this game of "Distraction". Don't you think your mother did this while she was pregnant with you? *Is it a boy or a girl? Is he/she going to be healthy? Will the birth go smoothly? Will there be complications? Will I be bedridden for months? What if the baby dies? What if it has a birth defect? What if it looks like my Uncle Leroy with the big ears and the wandering left eye?* And let's not give Mom all the credit. I'm sure Dad did his share of worrying, too. Am I right?

It's no surprise that we all learned to do the same thing — some of us more than others. My mother's side of the family is Jewish; my Dad's is Irish Catholic. Need I say more? Worrying, projecting, and compulsive daydreaming were an ever-present part of my growing up (and I'm not blaming my folks, because they grew up with the same). We realize it's insane and yet still we do it. Then we teach it to our kids.

This obsessive thought process is the Misery Conspiracy's way of distracting us from doing anything useful, while giving us the impression that somehow it will produce something of value. Ultimately, it just serves to keep us lost in our misery.

According to *A Course in Miracles,* the ego (our negative thought process) goes back and forth between grandiosity and littleness. "It is suspicious at best and vicious at worst," Marianne Williamson reminds us.

One minute, the Misery Conspiracy is telling you how great you are, giving you an inflated sense of self. "You are so much better than those other people," it claims. "Just wait 'til you hit the Big Time! Boy, will they be envious!"

Then, once your mind is filled with smug visions of material success, the ego turns around and rips the rug out from under you. "What is this garbage you've created? Pathetic! Who are you to think you can do this! You're not a professional. You don't have the credentials for this! Everyone will laugh at you. You'll go broke trying to sell it! What a naïve dreamer you are!"

What makes this such a successful game for the Misery Conspiracy is that it focuses your attention exclusively on the future with overtures of everything that ever went wrong for you in the past. It avoids the present the way a supermodel avoids a double bacon cheeseburger.

The past and the future are the Conspiracy's playground, and believe me, this playground is equipped with neurotic merry-go-rounds, obsessive-compulsive roller coasters, and sliding boards into Hell.

When we are caught up in the Conspiracy's way of thinking, we have no understanding of the present. But the present is the only place where anything exists. It is also the only place where you have the power to claim your Serenity and Joy. By obsessing over the past or future, you effectively lock yourself out of your Spiritual Home, completely forgetting where you hid the spare key. How brilliant is that? If only we could remember that we *are* the key, we wouldn't be standing around being miserable all the time.

Another version of the Conspiracy's game of "Distraction" includes luring you into tackling too many projects at once. For example, as an inspirational author and speaker, I catch myself filling my schedule with participation in all kinds of relevant organizations and activities. This has included voice lessons, Toastmasters, writers' groups, metaphysical discussion groups, women's spiritual circles, and more. Yikes!

It's amazing how little writing I get done when I have all these other things filling up my week. This serves the Misery Conspiracy well. If I never actually finish writing this book, then I don't have to deal with rejection letters from agents or publishers, much less negative reviews from critics. Safe from any potential rejection, I can wallow in a sea of incomplete projects and lukewarm self-loathing for not seeing them through. Fortunately, in the case of my book, I managed to break through the Conspiracy's distractions, because you're reading it.

The Conspiracy's game of "Distraction" also comes in another form; what I call "The Devil's in the Details." It is the obsession with minutiae that appear on the surface anyway to be important to a project. However, they only act as a delaying tactic.

If I've set aside time to write, I obsessively make sure I have the perfect background music to create the ideal ambiance to lure my Muse within striking distance.

Let's see, let me try some 80s rock. It's my favorite. A few songs later and... *Hmmmmm...no, the singing is distracting me from writing. I can't hear the words in my head that I want to write. Let's see, how about some smooth jazz. Yeah, that's the ticket. Another couple of songs later... No, still not the right music. Still too wordy and much too bouncy! Let me try some New Age.* A very long and mellow instrumental song later and... *zzzzzzzzzzzzzzzzzzzzzzzzzzzzzzzz.* Such are the distractions and delays of my minutiae-obsessed work process.

When I *really* want to write, it doesn't matter what's going on around me in terms of music or other background noise. I can write listening to New Age jazz or I can write in a noisy Starbucks ("Two-shot vanilla Americano with a shot of cold milk for Dharma"). I can and have written on a bouncy city bus weaving through rush-hour traffic on the freeway. I just ignore the rants of my negative thoughts telling me these aren't ideal conditions for writing the next inspirational bestseller, as if that has anything to do with my writing. All I need in order to write is to be willing to connect to the One Self.

Whatever direction your life's journey is going and whatever projects or activities seem meaningful to you, the Misery Conspiracy wants to keep you from them. It wants you miserable, after all. By focusing your attention on the past or on the future, the Conspiracy keeps you from being in the present moment, which is the only place you *can* be Happy. By distracting you with too many activities or with the minutiae of a single activity, your corrupted thought process prevents you from showing up in life, again blocking you from your Joy.

So how do we beat the Misery Conspiracy at its own game? If you really want to be Happy (and I'm guessing you do since you're still reading this book), then you must become aware of the times that your mind starts playing these games. Ask yourself from time to time, if you are enjoying what you are doing right now. Is your focus on what's going on this very moment? Are you in fact wandering off into the future or dredging up the past?

By remaining gently vigilant with our spiritual practice (something I talk about later on, so keep reading), we can stay on task and stay centered emotionally and spiritually. We are no longer thrown off balance by the wrong turns of the Misery Conspiracy. Sure, we can think about the future or reflect on the past now and then. But investing ourselves emotionally in anything not in the here-and-now robs us of our Joy.

Even in spiritual work like writing inspirational books, singing religious songs, or facilitating metaphysical discussion groups, the Misery Conspiracy likes to wreak havoc. Just because our activities are spiritual doesn't keep them out of the Conspiracy's reach.

In fact, the Conspiracy targets such activities for derailing, because not to do so would jeopardize its survival. When you connect with the One Self, you abandon all negative, ego thoughts. The Conspiracy of Misery collapses!

When you start feeling your emotions bouncing all over the place, take time to stop. Focus on your breathing for a few minutes. Tell yourself out loud, "I am willing to let go of this. I am willing to let go of results and just focus on the process!" Take time to pray, asking your personal Higher Power to guide you to a more stable way of thinking. Set aside at least fifteen minutes every morning to meditate, to allow your mind to *stop* thinking for a little while.

Don't play the Misery Conspiracy's "Distraction" game. It only serves to keep you off-balance and focused on what can't make you Happy. If you want to reclaim your Joy and Serenity, you must make other choices and use the tools that serve *your* goals of Happiness.

Chapter 3:
You Call That Happy?

What makes you Happy? A good movie? A gourmet meal? A nice glass of wine? Perhaps a good lover, or a beautiful sunset? Does holding a baby or petting a kitten make you Happy? Maybe listening to your favorite music or spending a day at the beach sparks your Happiness. I'm sure if I took a survey of a hundred people, and asked them what makes them Happy, I'd probably get a several hundred different responses. We all certainly have different tastes.

However, most of the things that we *think* make us Happy don't really make us Happy. They give us nothing more than a fleeting experience of pleasure, which is not the same as Happiness. However, the Misery Conspiracy would like us to think that pleasure *is* Happiness. In fact, the advertising world depends on you believing this. They use every trick in the book to make you think that whatever product or service they are selling will bring you Happiness. And like the mindless cattle that we too often are, we buy into it. Moooooo.

How many times have you said things like, "I'll be Happy when I get that promotion," or "If I could just meet the right guy or girl, it sure would make me Happy"? What about, "He makes me so mad," or "This job makes me so miserable." Whatever the object of our perceived Happiness or misery, it's all a big lie. The psychological name for it is "projection".

The best that any of these things can do is provide us with temporary pleasure or temporary unpleasantness. And then not long after finally getting whatever it is we are jonesing for, the pleasure fades and we're back to where we were before: feeling blah or dissatisfied, maybe even disappointed.

You would think that once this dissatisfaction sets in, we'd be on to the Misery Conspiracy's tricks. But no! The Conspiracy has that covered, too! Just as we're starting to feel the first twinges of remorse, realizing that what we were longing for didn't make us Happy after all, a new thought pops into our heads. "The next person or job or house or car or whatever will make us Happy." And because we're so accustomed to listing to that voice of lies, we believe it.

Now don't get me wrong. I have nothing against pleasure. Pleasure in moderation can be a wonderful thing. *However!* The Misery Conspiracy has an agenda and a very specific reason for keeping you focused on pleasure. If the Conspiracy can keep you chasing shadows, you won't bother looking for Happiness where it really exists. You remain blinded to the crazy dynamics that are sabotaging your Happiness.

My friend Marcus is like a little brother to me. He's about 10 years younger than I am, and a great guy. But like me at that age, he has a lot of issues that he's working through. One issue is that he keeps getting into relationships with people who are either emotionally unavailable, abusive or both. A lot of them have been alcoholics and drug addicts.

He doesn't understand why he keeps getting hooked up with people like this. When he does date these unhealthy women, it takes him a long time to admit that he's not getting his needs met in the relationship. He has to be taken to the cleaners financially or emotionally before he's finally willing to give up the doomed relationship.

Maybe the problem is that Marcus frequently smokes pot, gets drunk and occasionally does coke and ecstasy. No, he's *claims* not addicted! He just uses because it makes him Happy. When he said that, I responded, "You call that Happy?" He didn't understand.

The funny thing is that he dumped his last girlfriend because she had "a *serious* drug problem" that including running deliveries for a dealer. He also has had trouble holding on to a job for more than a month or two. With every job there is always a co-worker or supervisor with an attitude problem. Next thing you know, he's searching the want ads or calling the placement agency for another assignment.

I have no doubt that Marcus' drug use provides some temporary pleasure. But he clearly has no sense of Happiness, no lasting Joy, and certainly no Serenity. He calls me up every few weeks to fill me in on the latest list of lost jobs and dysfunctional girlfriends. He complains about how he misses his latest loser ex-girlfriend or he's excited about hooking up with either another ex or with some new chick he met (guess where?) at a rave, and that they only use *some of the time.*

It breaks my heart to hear how miserable he is and how he can never seem to catch a break. Marcus just can't see the connection between his drug use, the negative changes in his attitudes and behavior, and the never ending cycles of bad relationships and short-lived jobs. He resents the fact that his employers insist that he take a drug test. And he doesn't understand why all of the people he meets at raves and bars are dysfunctional, alcoholic drug users. All I can do is lovingly suggest that he be willing to see things differently, to see what dynamics are contributing to the circumstances of his life.

I want Marcus to be Happy. He's my semi-adopted little brother, after all. I want him to be able to enjoy life and experience total bliss the way that I have. But in order to do that, he has to choose Happiness over pleasure. He has to learn the lessons himself and make his own decision. And I truly believe that he eventually will. He's just going to have to get to the point where he's tired of substituting pleasure and misery for Joy and Serenity.

I have learned to enjoy all of the good things in my life. I appreciate my relationship with my partner. I appreciate being a writer. I am grateful that I can pay my bills (wasn't always the case). But none of that can make me Happy unless I choose to be Happy.

I recognize that my sense of Joy and Bliss come from within; from my deep spiritual connection to my Source and to you. And your joy comes from your connection to your Source and to me and everyone else in your life. Everything else is just frosting. Frosting is good, but I say let's eat the cake as well! Yum!

Chapter 4:
Matzoh Ball Soup for the Spirit

In addition to distracting us with meaningless images of past and future or with passing pleasures, the Misery Conspiracy uses our bodies to rob us of the Joy of Life, especially when we are ill or injured. It's very resourceful, this Misery Conspiracy. Through the subliminal societal messages (like advertising and infotainment), we have been conditioned to focus our attention on our physical discomforts, and away from the things that bring us Joy. The subtle, yet powerful, beliefs of the Misery Conspiracy equate us with our bodies and with being sick with suffering. None are true.

A few times a year, I manage to come down with a cold. With nose sore and running, eyes watering and body aching, I feel miserable when those microbes finally track me down. Of course, my addicted, codependent mind loves this because it's a great excuse to throw a pity party. It's as if my negative, loveless, victim-oriented thoughts are having a rave in my very congested body.

A Course in Miracles states that illness is a defense against the truth, that it is an attempt by our negative minds to prove to ourselves that we are vulnerable bodies living in a cruel and loveless world. Our emotional attachments to negative thought-patterns such as "I feel awful" and "No one understands how miserable I am" and "How will I ever get better?" are so strong that, in our insanity, we defend them at the obvious cost of our Peace of Mind.

To believe something other than this puts our whole world-view into jeopardy. It would suggest that we've been wrong about everything! And boy, do we hate being wrong! Such is our love/hate relationship with the Misery Conspiracy. We'd rather be miserable than actually admit we've made a mistake.

The truth is that you are not a body; and neither am I. Sure, we *have* bodies. We also may have cars, money, homes, and jobs, but we are not those, either. I did have a cousin Woodrow who thought he was a tree for about a year. We all just called him Woody. But I digress...

What we are is an integral part of the One Self. In other words, we are non-physical consciousness and energy, temporarily housed in a physical human form. We have the ability to manifest that energy into whatever form we choose to imagine. It is our minds, and not our bodies, that determine our reality. The cool thing about this is that as we let ourselves believe the Divine Truth of who we are, we don't feel so miserable.

If I have a cold, my nose may be runny and sore, but the experience of suffering can be lessened by my feelings of Serenity. We have the body experience (being sick), but this is separate from our mental experience of the body experience (being miserable about being sick). We tend to think of them as the same experience, but they're not.

Physical sensations aren't good or bad unless our minds assign them to such categories. Otherwise, they are just electro-chemical signals to our brains. The experience of "being sick" is just this. We habitually label these sensations as bad, but it doesn't have to be that way. All forms of suffering stem from this association. It is a decision (usually a subconscious one) we make — either, "I choose to be miserable because of these sensations" or "I choose to be at Peace regardless of these sensations." What we choose is ultimately what we experience. Which one do you prefer?

Another result of redirecting our thinking from a suffering mentality to Loving, Peaceful mindset is that we don't feel as vulnerable, weak or alone. We feel connected to the One Self. We feel loved and comforted. It doesn't matter what our bodies appear to be doing. It does matter what our minds are thinking. Imagine being Happy, even with a severe cold! That's better than a handful of antihistamines and it won't make you drowsy!

The root belief of the Misery Conspiracy is that all things end in misery; that misery is the ultimate truth. You've heard the phrase, "Life is pain?" Guess where that came from? Yep, the Misery Conspiracy!

When we let that be the guiding principle of our lives, we create and see a world of misery. But when we reject that belief and instead reconnect with the One Self, then we create and see a world where Love overwhelms lovelessness, and where Peace eliminates suffering.

What I find mind-blowing, and what I am still learning to trust, is that as we make a choice to be Happy, regardless of our physical experiences, our circumstances actually change for the better. The energy shifts and pulls in everything positive. Somehow our immune systems work more efficiently when we calm our minds. Studies have shown that people who laugh and have a positive outlook on life get sick less often and heal faster than those who choose to be miserable.

There is, of course, nothing wrong with taking medicine for illness. Believe me, when I start coming down with a cold, I pull out all the stops! I order two quarts of matzoh ball soup from Stan's Deli in Scottsdale (the best Jewish deli in Arizona, by the way). I grab the zinc lozenges, the Airborne, the Echinacea tea and 25-gallon drum of Nyquil. It serves no purpose, enlightened or otherwise, to force ourselves to suffer needlessly until we finally "get it." For now, take whatever medical steps the world of medicine would suggest, but at the same time work on realizing that none of this is any more than a manifestation of our collective thoughts.

As we continue working on our spiritual lessons, we no longer need the medicine. At some point in our spiritual development, we will simply see right through the Misery Conspiracy's false truths and instantly return to perfect health. Mind you, it may take some of us a few decades or a few millennia, but remember that, as eternal beings, we have all the time we need. You get the idea.

So next time you catch a cold, have some matzoh ball soup, plenty of orange juice, and maybe some cold medicine to help you sleep. But also take time to meditate as you are able. Repeat to yourself silently or aloud, "I am the expression of God's Love. I am the One Self." As you repeat it over and over, it will sink into your subconscious mind and you will feel better.

Chapter 5:
Hell For The Holidays

Now that I'm a spiritual guru, I never lose my cool. Any harsh words or unfortunate circumstances just roll off like rain off a duck's back. And if you believe any of this, I have some beachfront property in Tucson to sell you!

No, despite years of practice, my buttons get pushed every so often. It doesn't happen as often or severely as it used to. But it does happen. I hope I haven't totally ruined your perfect image of me.

The fact is that the effects of the Misery Conspiracy run deep. It takes times for us to uproot all of those negative thought patterns that we've spent a lifetime collecting. Fortunately, once we start on the road to spiritual recovery, we find a mental homing device that goes off when we get off track. I call this device the One Self. It's that gentle voice that says, "Hey, you! Is this really how you want to feel or are you open to alternatives?"

When I was growing up, the holidays were always insane. Our moderately dysfunctional family would naturally choose Thanksgiving, Christmas, and even Easter to turn up the crazy juices. Bickering, blaming, and gossiping were as plentiful as stuffing and cranberry sauce (you know, the jellied kind that makes a "thwok" sound when you get it out of the can).

These days, my nearest blood relative is more than 2000 miles away. While we are still learning to respect each other's chosen paths and eccentricities (no shortage of those in my family), this is a good, healthy distance. We call each other and talk about the weather without getting into our old crazy stuff, which is great progress for all of us. We can even fly out to visit each other every decade or so.

At times it still seems as if they are right here with me. Something will trigger me and I'll go back into my childhood-victim mindset, even if no one is actually victimizing me. Someone will say something, and I'm instantly projecting an entire drama in my head that has very little to do with the reality of the situation.

A few years ago, during the preparation of a Thanksgiving meal with my spouse, Eileen, and her parents, I lost my cool. As I was helping Eileen with the dinner rolls, she expected me to intuit exactly what she wanted me to do with them. As we were in my mother-in-law's kitchen, and I had no idea where anything was, I asked for clarification. However, her attention was focused on some other critical task that she was engaged in. She raised her voice. I raised my voice. Egos got triggered. Boom!

I went into the living room to sulk, an activity that I have perfected to an art form...okay, maybe something closer to finger-painting. Suddenly I was no longer in my in-laws' house in 2004. My mind had time warped back to my parents' or grandparents' house when I was a kid, where there was a lot of blaming and shaming all the time, especially during the holidays.

The Misery Conspiracy was in overdrive, telling me that I was stupid, worthless, etc. We all know the old tapes. And of course, I was blaming my partner for "making" me feel that way. *Poor me! The world just has no Compassion for pitiful old me.* Yeah, right! Dharma's pity party for one!

I sat in the living room marinating in my misery until we were called to dinner. Since I'm considered the "spiritual one" by Eileen and her parents, my mother-in-law always asks me to give the blessing. I wanted to say that I didn't feel like saying the blessing. I wanted to make a grand production about how unfairly Eileen had treated me. But something inside of me, that tiny ember of sanity said, "Dharma, you *need* to say the blessing; not for their sake, but for yours!"

So I said a short, but heartfelt blessing, which included, "Lord, open our minds to the awareness of Love's presence." It was that small, still voice speaking, the one that leads us out of insanity and into Peace. In that instant, I remembered that what I really wanted wasn't to be a "victim," but to be Happy. And suddenly, I found I could enjoy the meal.

It is rare that Eileen and I get upset with each other. I am grateful for that. Rarely have I seen a couple whose relationship works as well as ours. I am also grateful to have a chosen family who see something good in me that I sometimes am unable to see in myself. And finally, I am grateful to be able to learn when I bump up against my blocks — otherwise known as my "buttons" — to my awareness of Love's presence.

So yes, even after a decade in recovery, I still get triggered. I will probably get triggered when I have twenty or thirty years of recovery under my belt, although it will be even less frequent. Over time, though, as we pay attention to the dynamics and behaviors and feelings that we are experiencing, we learn to recognize the issues before we get triggered. We learn to walk around the pitfalls and eventually take a different route entirely. Our thought patterns gradually transform from focusing on the negative to focusing on the positive. And that, my friend, is precisely what Thanksgiving is all about. Well, that and going into a tryptophan coma after eating way too much turkey and dressing.

The next time the old Misery Conspiracy program gets you triggered, pay attention. Do your best to listen to what the One Self is saying to you. Sometimes it speaks just in your mind. Often it speaks through those around us, steering us back on track towards our goal of Happiness.

Chapter 6:
Divide and Conquer,
Then Divide and Conquer Again

One of the Misery Conspiracy's most destructive weapons is what I call the "us versus them" mentality. Behind every divorce, every war, every act of terrorism and every scalable wall on the United States - Mexico border (ladder not included) is this nasty salvo. The "us versus them" philosophy creates a false sense of worth and belonging (for "us") by designating certain other people ("them") as the "real cause" of our problems. All it really accomplishes is to turn *us* against *them*, making *everybody* miserable.

What amazes me is how "us versus them" doesn't stop with dividing a group into two subgroups. It then works to divide the subgroups into sub-subgroups, and the sub-subgroups into sub-subsubgroups, and the...oh, heck, you get the idea. Over time "them" gets larger and larger, while "us" whittles down to no one. Pretty soon, we find we have isolated ourselves from everyone else. To paraphrase Marianne Williamson, when someone tells you, "It's you and me against the world," it's time to switch sides!

I have seen this even in the unlikeliest of places: the GLBT (gay, lesbian, bisexual, and transgender) community. One would think that a community that embraces diversity would be immune from the "us versus them" mentality. For the most part, that is the case. But as a gay pastor once told me, "We're all about diversity until we meet someone that's *really* diverse."

There is a broad sense of cohesion in the GLBT community. But it's not hard to find those who think certain segments of the community don't belong and should be voted off the island. Those that blend in well with the straight community ("straight acting gays" or SAGs) have historically complained about their more flamboyant brothers and sisters (drag queens, dykes on bikes, leathermen, etc.).

According to the SAGs, the queens and the diesel dykes are making it harder for the GLBT community to be accepted by the public at large. And of course, the more flamboyant crowd has often accused the SAGs of kowtowing to the homophobic extremists.

Years ago, there was a woman who attended a (predominantly lesbian) women's music festival in the Midwest. She discovered the hard way about how intolerant some people can be. For the first day of the three-day festival, she enjoyed the music and the camaraderie of her fellow women. But then one of the more militant lesbian attendees began to suspect that this woman had not been born a woman. When confronted, the woman admitted that she was a post-op transsexual, but that now she was physiologically female.

This revelation of honesty became the spark for a confrontation. The woman was forced to leave the festival, not even allowed to gather her belongings. The woman was hurt and humiliated by people that she had trusted to stand for openness and diversity.

To add insult to injury, the organizers of the festival responded not by condemning this act of ignorance and intolerance, but by endorsing it. The next year, they proudly stated that the festival was for "womyn [sic] born womyn only"! And we wonder where people get the image of lesbians as "femi-nazis"? It's from people who fall prey to the "us versus them" mentality and who follow the Misery Conspiracy's order to divide and conquer, and then divide and conquer again!

To their credit, the transgender community and its supporters now host their own festival called "Camp Trans" right across the street from the trans-phobic one, creating not only a trans-friendly alternative, but bringing attention to the issue of discrimination within the ranks of the GLBT community. Rock on!

In every society, every religion, every social group, there is the idea of "them". *They are the enemy! They are the problem! They are the evil-doers! They are stupid! They are corrupt! I can't be Happy if they are around or are in power or have something that I don't have! We have to stop them! We have to take what's theirs and make it ours! We have to kill them!*

My friend Michelle is a big fan of Air America, a progressive talk radio network. When she first told me about the emerging network, I was excited because I was tired of all of the one-sided, narrow-minded propaganda put out by the likes of Bill O'Reilly and Rush Limbaugh. "Finally," I thought, "we can have talk shows that present a more balanced, more honest view without all of the name-calling that is so common in right-wing talk shows." I was wrong.

When I listened to some of Air America's shows, I found the same kind of semi-accurate, one-sided mudslinging, only this time, the mud was coming from the other direction. The blame was the same. Only the "them" had changed. I was really disappointed. I had expected more from Air America. Thank goodness I still have NPR.

While I agree that the Bush Administration has been rife with corruption, egomania, stray birdshot, and very, very poor judgment, calling them the "Bush crime family" is a bit much. Talking only about what the Republicans are doing wrong (which admittedly is a LOT) and not saying what the Democrats had been doing (either right or wrong), is not all that impressive. Mud is mud. Propaganda is still propaganda, no matter which way it's spun.

As hard as it is to admit sometimes (even for me), the truth is that there is no "them". It's all "us". We are all human. We all want to be Happy. We all want to have a safe place to live and raise our families. We all want to have access to healthy food, clean water, and a community that supports us in becoming the best that we can be. The Democrats want this, and so do the Republicans and Independents and Libertarians and members of the

Green Party. Israelis want this and so do Palestinians and Iraqis and Iranians and North Koreans and South Koreans.

The only problem is that some of "us" make poor choices in how to best accomplish these goals. The solution is to lovingly help those of us making the poor choices to make better, more loving choices.

One of the big topics these days is illegal immigration. In my home state of Arizona, it's a BIG topic. There's a lot of talk about how *they* are robbing Americans of jobs, and how *they* drain money away from public education and healthcare. Other people complain that illegal immigrants are criminals and possibly terrorists. I even heard one acquaintance complain that they were stealing his scholarships that he "worked so hard for". I doubt he worked much harder than immigrant student that was awarded the scholarship (who had to learn English on top of learning the subject matter itself).

This is classic Misery Conspiracy thinking about how "they" are the problem. "Us versus them" focuses on limited resources and is founded on the belief that in order for you to have something, you must take it away from someone else. But these are all lies. Nowhere in all of these loveless excuses for xenophobia is there any consideration for what the undocumented immigrant has already been through to get here or what they could contribute to our society if given the opportunity. That's because the Misery Conspiracy just wants to keep us miserable. And one way of doing this is by dividing our world into "us and them".

Every culture has a word to describe "the outsider". Some have several words for it, most of which have a negative connotation. Isn't it interesting how words like "savage", "alien", "gringo", "gaijin", "infidel", "goyim", "heathen", "faggot", etc., all convey a sense of unworthiness. We think that because *they* are different from *us*, that *they* aren't worth loving or respecting.

I once heard a joke that demonstrated the tragic silliness of this divisive philosophy. In fact, I've heard several versions of it, only with different groups mentioned. Here's the joke:

A man arrived at the Pearly Gates of Heaven
and was escorted around Heaven by Saint Peter.

The man was shown choruses of angels singing praises and songs of joy. He was shown the streets of gold and all the treasures of Heaven. He was even re-united with his deceased friends and relatives. The man was overjoyed with how wonderful Heaven was.

Then the man looked off into the distance and saw this small group of people all huddled together. The man turned to Saint Peter and asked, "Who's that group of people way out there?"

Saint Peter chuckled. "Oh, *them*? They are the [fill in the blank with the divisive religious group of your choice]. They think they are the only ones here."

When we get it in our head that there are people who aren't worth respecting, who aren't worth understanding, who aren't worth loving, then we become the ones who are isolated. We shut ourselves off from all of that is good and beautiful in our lives and in our lives to come.

I have found that even with my years of teaching spiritual dynamics, I have to be constantly vigilant for this weapon of the Misery Conspiracy. All it takes is someone to say something that is outrageously unkind and narrow-minded and I feel this need to make that person a "them". *They are so full of crap! How can they say something like that? They are so stupid! Someone should get rid of them!*

To deal with this, I have to use several tools in my spiritual toolbox to stop my mind from judging whoever is pushing my buttons. These include brief prayers for Divine guidance, a willingness to see them differently, letting go of my loveless thoughts, and remembering the principle of love ("the love I withhold from anyone, I withhold from myself"). Pre-emptive measures such as daily meditation time, reading spiritual literature and spending time helping others also helps to curb this inclination.

Don't let the Misery Conspiracy rob you of your Joy by engaging in the "us versus them" mentality. Remember that *they* are not the enemy. *They* are just doing the best that *they* can with what *they* have, and often what *they* have is the poison fed to *them* for years by the Misery Conspiracy and by *us*. The enemy is never *them* because there is no *them*. *They* are an essential part of *us*. Our real enemy is always hate, fear and all forms of lovelessness. Fight the Conspiracy! Love those who drive you nuts!

Chapter 7:
Guilty Out of the Gate? Oh, Please!

When I was in my early 20's, I was taught the concept of "original sin." Boy, was that a creation of the Misery Conspiracy! It's a philosophy filled with messages like, "God hates you" and "You are guilty." It is a belief designed to strip you of your power and rob you of your Joy in the glorious name of religiosity. But there is a way to rework this concept, so that it serves the purposes of the One Self (i.e., to help you reclaim your Joy and Peace) instead of the Conspiracy.

As it was explained to me at the time, original sin means that every person is condemned to Hell by God from the moment of birth. The rationale (and I use the term loosely) for this automatic Divine Rejection lies with the belief that Adam and Eve screwed up (the original sin), and then passed their guilt on to us. What a classic case of guilt by association! Clearly this idea that the whole of humanity is inherently guilty and unloved by God is a concept created and perpetuated by the Misery Conspiracy.

Oddly enough, advocates of this guilt-at-birth belief defend it zealously, at the expense of their own Peace of Mind. "God said it (He didn't), I believe it (they *really* do), and that settles it!" That's their philosophy, and they are certainly entitled to it. Personally, I think such an attachment to guilt is incredibly sad.

As far as the guilt-at-birthers are concerned, if we weren't all guilty, then Jesus' death on the cross would lose its meaning. Their whole understanding of God, Life and the Universe would be called into question. As someone who has been through that (because I used to believe it myself), I can attest that such a radical paradigm shift is a scary thing to experience! The possibility of a more enlightened, less bloodthirsty take on the whole crucifixion/resurrection deal is a ticking time bomb that threatens the Universe of Guilt they hold so dear.

It makes no sense that the Children of God, created by God and in the likeness of God, would then be condemned by God right out of the chute. But that's the religion of the Misery Conspiracy. The innocent are guilty!

When we pull back enough to really see the dynamics of this philosophy, it makes God look like La Llorona, the legendary mother who kills her children out of grief or regret. It does not sound like the Divine Presence of Love. What kind of parent kicks their child out of the house for making a mistake or even acting defiant?

Let me suggest an alternative theory. Rather than Jesus dying to pay for our spiritual debts, what if the whole crucifixion and resurrection deal was to teach us that we *have* no spiritual debts? Remember Jesus' parable of the Prodigal Son? What was the father's response to his son upon his return?

Did the father (option A) condemn his prodigal son to be tortured indefinitely to pay for his mistakes? Or did he (option B) kill his "obedient" son to atone for the sins of the prodigal son? Or did he (option C) rejoice at the safe return of his son, welcoming him home with open arms and throwing a celebration in his honor?

Okay, have you guessed? The correct answer is option C. The father rejoiced at the safe return of his son, welcoming him home with open arms and throwing a celebration in his honor. Did you get it right? Awesome! Thank you for playing "Jesus Jeopardy"!

And what can we learn from this? This isn't a story about a father kicking a disobedient child out of the home. It's about a child who runs away and then returns to find a grateful and welcoming father. God isn't looking to punish us for our mistakes. He just wants us to get out of the predicament that we created for ourselves and come Home.

The truth is that we, as the Divine Children of God, are innocent. We make mistakes, but they're not who we are. They have no bearing on our innocence. We simply don't understand the Truth. If we really had a clue about what's going on, we would never think or behave the way we do. It follows, then, that God *never* withheld His Love from us, any more than any decent parent would stop loving a child for reaching for a hot stove or soiling a diaper.

We, on the other hand, have blocked our awareness of the All-Loving One Self. In our insanity, through our judgments of ourselves and others, we have lost touch with our Source. When we withhold Love for any reason, we withhold it from ourselves and we block our awareness of God's Love.

That being said, there is a more enlightened version of the "original sin" concept. The word "sin" was originally an archery term meaning "missed the mark." Therefore, the "original sin" was the first time our thinking missed the mark; our first loveless thought. From that loveless thought came our experience of lovelessness, fear, and guilt. Jesus' purpose was not to suffer for our guilt, but to help us realize that we simply aren't guilty. Jesus came to correct our thinking and restore us to Love, Peace and communion with each other and with God.

The Misery Conspiracy's version of "original sin" claims to eradicate guilt, but it doesn't. Even if Jesus' execution got us out of the doghouse with God (according to this twisted logic), we still feel guilty that we needed Jesus to suffer horribly and die, just so we could go to Heaven. That doesn't alleviate guilt, it magnifies it! It's a classic Conspiracy switcheroo!

The enlightened version, however, shows us where our thinking went wrong, the point at which our thoughts diverged from those of the One Self and everything literally went to Hell! It then redirects us to the Light. It helps us refocus on Love, Compassion, and Forgiveness.

When we become willing to let go of our unloving thoughts (especially the ones that focus on guilt), and begin to listen to the Voice of the One Self that speaks to each one of us, "original sin" is reversed because the error in our thinking is corrected. Repenting of our sins means nothing more than turning back (repenting) from our errors (sins) in thinking. When we do this, all of the negative drama, guilt and pain vanish, restoring us to Peace and Joy.

What I want you to take away from this chapter more than anything else is the need to re-examine your current belief systems, especially if they were spoon-fed to you as a child. Put them to the test.

Do they alleviate guilt or magnify it? Do they celebrate your inherent worth, or emphasize your inadequacies? Even Buddha told his followers to put his teachings to the test. Be wary of any doctrine or dogma that discourages questioning. If it does, odds are it comes straight from the Misery Conspiracy.

Chapter 8:
Duh!

It continues to amaze me how subtle and sneaky the Misery Conspiracy is. One would think (at least I do) that someone, who has studied spiritual dynamics for years would be free of all prejudices, particularly the ones based on religious or political beliefs. One would think that, and one would be wrong.

Like the Bermuda grass in my backyard that refuses to die, my insane little thought system continues to creep in to judge others, project guilt, and justify my resentments, even on issues I claim to be open-minded about. Sure, I don't do it as much as I used to, but I still do it. I've just learned to cover my tracks better.

One time, the nastiness that is the Misery Conspiracy sneaked in as I was commenting on someone's blog, presumably in the spirit of ministry. This blogger had values and political views quite different from mine. She is a conservative Christian Republican, whereas I tend to be more liberal on most issues.

Normally, I have a lot of respect for differing viewpoints, including those of the Conservative Right. I don't agree with them, but I respect the rights of those who do. This blogger, however, managed to find my hot buttons and give them a good whack! Her blog postings suggested that anyone who isn't white, heterosexual, wealthy, American (natives only!), a born-again Christian and an unflagging supporter of the Bush administration didn't deserve to have any rights. She was clearly a devout follower of the Misery

Conspiracy in my mind. Unfortunately, my response wasn't any more enlightened.

In my comment to her posting, I pointed out how judgmental she was towards people who are different. I took great pride (big, BIG mistake) in dissecting her political and religious attitudes, explaining how un-Christ-like they were. I quoted Scripture and referenced solid historical facts. I built a magnificent case (at least to my triggered, holier-than-thou mind), leading to the ultimate conclusion that she was an evil hypocrite unworthy of Love or understanding. Can you say "projection"?

Now, who was the devout follower of the Misery Conspiracy? Yes, that would be me: Little Miss Can't-Be-Wrong. In spite of all my studies and practice of letting go of judgment and loveless thoughts, here I was slamming this woman. Not just her blog or her opinions — I was condemning her!

By the grace of all that is Divine, I took the time to re-read what I had written before saving it. I suddenly saw what I was really doing. Duh! I wasn't shining the Light of Spirit. I wasn't extending Love. My ego was in full, turbocharged grandiosity mode. I was trying to *appear* holy and enlightened, but really all I was doing was bashing her. I wasn't trying to demonstrate and teach Love. I was trying to put her in her place.

Fortunately, I deleted my comments before posting them. Then I asked my Higher Power to change my thinking, to help me see this person in a more loving way. It's amazing what miracles such willingness produces, isn't it? Admittedly it's not quite as impressive as parting a large body of water or feeding multitudes with a basket of food (a miracle I leave up to the local food bank), but such a change in attitude from resentment to Love is a true miracle. It won't get me canonized as a saint, but it certainly made me feel better.

Instead of a rant, I simply wrote, "I love you. Be careful of judging people. You will lose your sense of Peace. God wishes you Peace, Joy and Love, as do I. God bless."

There really isn't anything else I needed to say. It's not my job to force her to change her views or to make her feel like a jerk for judging people outside of her circle. I just need to Love her.

Be vigilant for the tricks of the Misery Conspiracy. The Bible describes it as "a roaring lion looking for someone to devour." It's not outside us, as some people would have you believe. It *is* us, and it's amazing how subtle and clever we can be, even if we are only outwitting ourselves. Listen to what you think and say. Don't rob yourself of your Peace.

Chapter 9:
Monkey Bait

Attachments! They are the glue that holds us in the grip of the Misery Conspiracy! No, I'm not talking about the files you electronically paperclip to your emails. I'm talking about the emotional attachments we have to things and people and ideas that drag us down when Life doesn't go our way. Our attachments to our spouse or our utterly unsatisfying job or simply our need to be right snare us like a prey animal, even as misery approaches with arrows and spears and curare-tipped blow darts.

Did you know that in the Amazon rainforests of South America, monkeys are considered good eating by certain native tribes? Yeah, I know, not exactly what I call good eating. But when you live in the Amazon, you eat what's available, including monkeys.

Monkeys, however, live high in the trees and move quickly. That makes them hard to catch. But the local hunters have developed a way to make catching them a bit easier (good for the hunters, bad for the monkeys).

The hunters hollow out a gourd and create a small hole in the side. Into this they put some fruit or rice or something else that monkeys like to eat. They then attach this baited gourd securely to a tree and wait. Eventually, a monkey comes along, smells the food inside the gourd and reaches in to grab it.

The catch is that the hole in the gourd is just barely large enough for the average adult monkey to squeeze its empty hand through. It is *not* large enough, however, for the monkey to pull out its hand while holding the piece of fruit. In order to withdraw its hand, the monkey must let go of the fruit...or find a monkey with really small hands, I guess.

This is where things get bizarre. When the hunter shows up, the monkey must choose between holding onto the fruit inside the gourd or saving its life by releasing the fruit and escaping into the canopy of the trees. You would think that the monkey would value its life more than getting that piece of fruit. That, however, is not the case. The hunters have found that the monkey will scream and hop around, all the while keeping itself trapped by holding onto the fruit. Thus, the foolish monkey is easily killed by the hunter.

Sadly, we humans aren't that much brighter than monkeys. Sure, we wear clothes, drive cars and some of us even know how to program our digital video recorders. But when it comes to finding Peace of Mind, we often haven't a clue! We are so easily tempted by the Misery Conspiracy's loveless thought process that we cling to it for dear life, all the while denying ourselves our God-given right to Joy and Peace of Mind.

In a lot of ways, we are like those monkeys with their hands stuck in the gourd, hopping around shouting, "I'm trapped! I'm trapped!" Okay, monkeys can't talk, but if they could, that's what they'd be shouting. I'm sure of it.

Once I was speaking to my friend, Michelle, who had been having a conflict with her co-worker, Pat. Apparently, Pat had been on a three-month campaign at the office to undermine and discredit Michelle, which included trying to take over some of Michelle's job responsibilities. Pat had also been bad-mouthing Michelle in front of co-workers. After a few months of Pat's hostile behavior, Michelle's emotions and her ability to focus at work began to suffer.

I asked Michelle how she had responded to Pat's maneuvering and backstabbing. Michelle replied that she had discussed the situation several times with the general manager and had brought up the issue during manager meetings, which both she and Pat attended. Fortunately, upper management saw through Pat's disruptive and childish actions and reprimanded her. Unfortunately, Pat was a determined little corporate climber and continued her attempts to manipulate her way into Michelle's job.

Michelle continued to complain to upper management about Pat's ongoing passive-aggressive behavior. And Pat would be reprimanded again. I could tell from the tone of Michelle's voice that she got some pleasure in successfully and repeatedly putting Pat in her place. Still, the situation had regressed to the point that the very thought of Pat would upset Michelle.

The conflict between the two of them continued to escalate. Michelle's focus at work revolved more and more around Pat and less about her own work responsibilities. *What is Pat going to pull today? She's such a jerk. How can I stop her from stealing my power? How can I get her fired?*

I empathize with Michelle's upset feelings. No one likes to be the target of an office bully, which Pat undoubtedly was. At the same time, how we see a situation like this can greatly affect whether we get upset or keep our Serenity. It can also influence (though not necessarily control) whether the situation continues or gets resolved.

Even in situations where we are in the right, we can't control other people. Believe me, before I got sober I was a master manipulator and it nearly cost me my life. We can have influence, but never control.

By choosing love over hate, we can also alter the dynamic of a situation and, at the very least, no longer lose our sense of Peace, no matter what the other person does. When we value Serenity over control, the crisis always seems to resolve itself. It's bizarre how it works, but after years of practicing this, I know it's true.

Michelle certainly had a right to be upset with Pat's hostile behaviors. At the same time, she also had a right to be Happy. Which "right" she chose to exercise was entirely her decision. Similarly, you have the right to be angry or sad or frustrated or depressed about situations in your life. And just like Michelle, you also always, *always* have the right to be Happy in spite of what's going on. What you experience (upset or Joy) is entirely dependent upon whichever one you value most.

We tend to think we need a tangible reason to be Happy. *I need to have all my bills paid to be Happy. I need to be married. I need to be single. I need to have a better job. I need to have more kids. I need to have fewer kids. I need to drive a faster car. I need to have 24-hour maid service, and a butler and a pool boy who wears only a Speedo at all times.*

We believe that if things are not going well for us (i.e. every need, want and whim gets met right now), we can't possibly be Happy. Even if most things are going well for us, we'll still focus on the few issues that aren't going so well. This is a classic example of fear-based or ego-based thinking. It is the Misery Conspiracy in action. The good news is that we have the power to overcome it.

It helps to look a little deeper at a situation. Let's take the case of a bully (be it on the playground, the workplace or even a terrorist). Look at the bully's motivations. Why do people attack other people? There really is only one answer: fear. You can dress it up as revenge or meanness or the will of God or a bad childhood or a dysfunctional marriage or Italian shoes that are a size and a half too tight. Underneath the window dressing, it's just fear.

Clearly, Pat has a low self-image. In order to cope with her lack of Love towards herself, she attacks those around her like a wounded animal. When Michelle retaliated, it reinforced Pat's loveless thoughts. Is it any surprise then that the conflict escalated?

Imagine what would have happened if Michelle had chosen to respond with Compassion instead of retaliating with the same lovelessness that Pat was projecting. What if Michelle had gone up to Pat and said, "Pat, I really care about you, but I'm concerned about your behavior. What's this really about? How can we resolve this conflict?" If Michelle had done this, the probability of a peaceful resolution would have dramatically increased.

When we favor our right to be upset over our right to be Happy, we're just like the monkey clinging to the fruit inside the gourd trap. It might be sweet fruit. It might be tasty fruit. But it's not worth the price we pay to hold onto it. Unless the monkey releases the bait and scampers away, he's going to be the guest of honor at the village's next feast.

Our right to be upset is what I call "monkey bait." It's so tempting. And revenge seems so sweet, especially when it is so richly deserved. It's hard to let go of it, yet at the same time, it's killing us — robbing us of the freedom we deserve.

The next time someone pushes your button, remember "monkey bait." Remember that while you have a right to be upset, you also have a right to be Happy. You can get mad or you can blow it off and say, "Whatever!" and bless whoever pushed your buttons. Don't let "monkey bait" keep you trapped in fear and misery.

Ask yourself what you have emotional attachments to. What situations or objects seem so important to you that their loss would leave you devastated? The Misery Conspiracy tells you that these are the things that make you Happy. But there is nothing outside of you that can make you Happy. Happiness comes from within. It comes from realizing who you are, recognizing your beauty and worth, and sharing it with the world.

Chapter 10:
How Much Does Shame Suck?!

"Live never to be ashamed if anything you say or do is published, even if what is published is not true." Richard Bach, *Illusions*

This is my favorite quote from *Illusions*. It speaks to a culture obsessed with guilt, shame and appearances; a culture ruled by the Misery Conspiracy. How many careers and lives have been ruined by slanderous news stories, whether the allegations were true or not? The Western media makes billions of dollars a year on such stories because they sell. It's as if we can't get enough of this kind of news.

The media isn't the only organization that uses this game of shame. Many political and religious organizations have used shame (and the consequences it brings) as a source of power to control the masses. When I came out of the closet, my mother's biggest concern was what the neighbors were going to think. Shame *seems* to be a very powerful weapon for the Misery Conspiracy.

I emphasize the word "seems" because shame only has the power we give it. It can control us only if we buy into its flawed logic. There really is no reason to be ashamed. I mean it. It serves absolutely no purpose but to make us miserable.

I've made a lot of mistakes in my time. I've hurt people. I've blown opportunities. I've been a drunk and a manipulator. I've done a lot of stupid things. But then, we've all done stupid things. And I would venture to say most of us have hurt others in some fashion. It's part of being human. When we recognize this and are unafraid to allow others see our humanity, shame loses its power over us.

Shame isn't what turns us around. Neither is guilt. We may experience shame at the point that we've recognized our errors, but it's not what drives us. It is only the deep spiritual realization that our thoughts and behaviors no longer serve our needs that makes us change. We see that the needs and feelings of others have some importance, and eventually realize that these needs are just as important as our own.

More often than not, shame keeps us trapped in addictive or compulsive behaviors. Shame easily creates a cycle of "acting out" (drinking, drugging, controlling, violence, etc.), followed by regret, then shame, then a desperate need to alleviate the guilt, which typically leads back to more acting out. Those of us who are addicts or codependents realize that our acting out is nothing more than an attempt to deal with unpleasant feelings. Chief among these feelings is shame.

It is the recognition of this truth that makes Alcoholics Anonymous and other 12-step programs work so well. Everyone at the meetings is a drunk or an addict. No one is better than anyone else, making it easier to share our stories without feelings of guilt.

Before AA was formed, alcoholics were considered hopeless cases. No amount of psychotherapy seemed to help. Alcoholics, as a rule, have a hard time connecting with therapists on a deeply spiritual level. Unless the therapist has struggled personally with the demons of addiction, there is an inequality that makes it difficult for the alcoholic to break through the wall of shame. Trust is nearly impossible.

In the circles of AA, there is no inequality. All of us have the same problem. We are powerless over our drug of choice, whether it's alcohol, meth, or unhealthy relationships. Our lives are in ruins or at least on the verge of collapse. A bond is created among those who attend, alleviating enough of the shame to allow the healing to begin.

At an Al-Anon meeting, someone once told me, "What somebody thinks or says about you is none of your business." This is very consistent with Richard Bach's quote. At the time, my response was, "What do you mean it's none of my business? Of course, it's my business! They're talking about me!"

Many years of recovery later, I realized that what that person said was true. Our business isn't what someone thinks, says, or writes about us. Our business is what *we* think, say, or write about *them* and ourselves. Of course, most of us would rather complain about what other people are doing, instead of looking at what we are doing. It's another example of the Misery Conspiracy at work.

Once I was walking around downtown Phoenix. I came to an intersection and had to wait for the light to change before crossing the street. While I was waiting, I noticed that a shabbily dressed guy on the other side was screaming obscenities. Then I realized that I was the one he was shouting these obscenities at. As far as I knew, I had never encountered this man in my life. I crossed the street in the other direction and avoided him in case he got violent.

When I mentioned the incident to one of my co-workers at City Hall, she replied, "Oh, that's Crazy Larry! He does that to people all the time. Don't worry. He shouts a lot, but he's harmless. And it's not really directed at you. He's just in a different world."

When my suspicions of Crazy Larry's schizophrenia were confirmed, I realized that his rants were nothing to be offended about, as his tortured mind was projecting his craziness onto the world he saw. Yes, he called me "bitch" several times (about the only word of his I can print), but he clearly wasn't in touch with the reality of who I am. So what did it matter what he thought?

We only get upset at someone else's negative opinions of us if we share those negative opinions of ourselves or suspect they may be true. If we didn't agree with what the other person said, we would just blow it off as a ridiculous notion or the rantings of a lunatic. After all, who cares what crazy people think of us if we know they're wrong?

Our fear of change, our addiction to shame, and most of all the fear that we aren't the poor, innocent victims we pretend to be all conspire together in our minds to keep us victimized and powerless. It's really sick because we do it to ourselves. And yet, as I learned when I began working on my recovery, change isn't as scary as we make it out to be.

Letting go of our shame, even if we have made mistakes, frees us up to reclaim our personal power and Serenity. As for giving up our identity as the Universe's victim, it's really not the cool gig that we thought it was when we signed up for it.

Of course, one caveat to all of this is that when several people are sending you the same message, it can be beneficial to at least consider what they are saying. For example, my friend Marcus has had several relationships go sour over the past few years. Some of these ended with his ex-girlfriends accusing him of passive aggressive and violent behavior (one even got a restraining order against him).

Marcus denied any form of physical or verbal violence, and in my own experience, I have never seen him behave violently towards me or anyone else. Marcus dismisses these claims as his ex-girlfriends projecting their own baggage onto him, which for all I know could be the case.

However, he did grow up with a violent, rage-aholic father. He also uses drugs occasionally. I suspect that there may be more to the story than what he has shared with me or admitted to himself. I have seen rage-aholics focus their violence on a single person (usually a love interest or family member), while the rest of the world sees only their docile, friendly side. My point is that when several people you know personally accuse you of a certain type of behavior, you might want to look into that.

Getting back to the original focus of this chapter, the Misery Conspiracy wants you to be ashamed of who you are, what you've done, or what some people *think* you have done. Shame is used by a variety of power structures to "keep you in line" and to keep you weak. This need not be the case.

When we let go of the shame placed on us by an insane world, we gain a better understanding of what our worth really is and where we need to grow. When we focus our efforts on being loving and compassionate towards others, we no longer worry about what other people say or think about us. Instead, we can see any accusations as someone else's drama.

So let us live our lives free of shame, regardless of what anyone else says or thinks. Let us let go of our attachment to their opinions. Let us let go of our own negative opinions of ourselves and others. And let us live with such Love and Compassion that the world will see our true worth.

Section Two:
Lessons Learned
the Hard Way

Chapter 11:
The Worst Things I Love About Retreats

Life is a wondrous thing. It has the incredible capacity to teach us what we most need to learn, including how to defeat the Misery Conspiracy. Mind you, these lessons don't always come labeled as lessons. Often they come disguised as tragedies, frustrations, annoying people and disappointments. But this mis-labeling is actually helpful, because it serves to throw the Misery Conspiracy off-balance. Remember that the Misery Conspiracy is very clever. Often it takes a Love lesson dressed up as a disaster to sneak in under the radar before we will let go of our misery.

In the autumn of 2005, I went on an overnight women's retreat in Payson, Arizona. For those not familiar with this small city, Payson is located in the northern part of Arizona, nestled in mountains covered with ponderosa pine, juniper and a sprinkling of hardwood trees. Not only is it a great place for a women's retreat, it is also a blissful escape from the desert heat of Phurnace (I mean, *Phoenix*), Arizona.

Retreats can be wonderful experiences. I have attended quite a few in my four decades on this planet, including women's retreats, youth retreats, meditation retreats, and even solo retreats. I keep going on these excursions with the expectation that, at last, I will find the answers that have been escaping me all these years. I will experience that Great Spiritual Epiphany where I become an Enlightened Master! At the very least, I hope for some much needed Peace and quiet. But, as we say in AA, expectations are premeditated resentments.

For this women's retreat in Payson, I was asked to give one of the talks, and not just any talk. I was chosen to give "The Bonfire Talk". Pretty impressive, huh? I chose "Finding Peace through Forgiveness" as my subject matter; a topic I felt I had pretty much mastered.

As I prepared for the retreat, I had this romantic vision of giving my talk at the bonfire, with everyone listening intently, *quietly* sipping hot cocoa, and gaining great insights from the sharing of my wisdom. This vision was undoubtedly a setup from the Misery Conspiracy, because the reality was nothing like that. Big surprise!

From the moment I started speaking to the group nestled around the bonfire, the distractions began. First, small groups of people kept coming from the cabins to sit by the fire (chatting and laughing as they found their seats), while others kept going back for hot cocoa or gloves or the flashlight buried in their pack. This went on for a while. But being the wise woman that I am (tongue planted firmly in cheek), I *tried* to ignore them.

As the fire began to burn down, one of the women started throwing more wood onto it. Every time she did, it sent a spray of sparks towards the other women, causing them to shriek in panic. Still others hollered every time the wind shifted and blew smoke in their direction. By the end of my talk on Forgiveness and finding Peace, even I was struggling to feel Peaceful, much less forgiving.

There were other ego-triggering events at the retreat. During someone else's presentation, a carload of late arrivals burst in waving, hugging, and shouting "hey" to people across the room. That presenter soon exacted her revenge by getting passive aggressive with one of the late arrivals, shaming her for not engaging in the same religious practice as herself.

Later that afternoon, one of the organizers barked orders at the women to set a table for everyone, rather than politely asking for their help. "What are you people doing just sitting there? Put that table cloth on the table! Move those paper plates! Wash that pot!" Good thing her cooking was better than her attitude!

For a women's spiritual retreat, it seemed infused with an awful lot of unspiritual behavior. I left there feeling disappointed and triggered instead of Peaceful and renewed. Not even the idyllic surroundings of Payson could compete with the insanity we brought with us.

So was the retreat a failure? Not at all! As with nearly every retreat I've attended, including my solo retreats, this one presented a microcosm of the human condition. No matter where we go, there we are, dragging our quirks, pet peeves, judgments, assumptions and, let's not forget, expectations.

We bring all of our emotional and spiritual baggage with us, even 5,000 feet above sea level. But this is not a bad thing. These are the issues we need to work on. This is where the real insights of the retreats come from; not from the talks, not from the hikes, not from the beauty of nature, not even from the group meditations. They come from learning to deal with the crap of life!

When we go on a spiritual retreat, expecting God to just download enlightenment into our brainpans, we are going to be sorely disappointed. Even if we get to feeling really great at the retreat, we eventually go home and the same old stuff starts up again. Family members and bosses demand unreasonable amounts of our time. Things break. People are rude. Within a week, the Serenity of the retreat has vanished.

For my money, the most effective retreats are the ones where our egos get triggered and we have the awareness to say, "God, I'm upset right now. Help me let go of my judgments and resentments." Real enlightenment comes from the recognition of our shortcomings and the willingness to ask for Divine guidance to change. These are the lessons that bring Peace, not only at the retreat, but in the real world as well. This is how we overthrow the Misery Conspiracy and turn the world into a place of Joy and Serenity.

So the next time you go on a retreat, or even to a family reunion or on vacation to some tropical destination, pay attention to what triggers you, ask for Divine help, and then be willing to see things differently. This is where you will discover the true gifts and lessons that a retreat can offer.

Chapter 12:
Jumping Off of a Perfectly Good Cliff

Remember all those lessons you were taught in school — everything from the laws of geometry to who fought the French and Indian War (I still can't remember)? Out of all that you were taught, how much of it have you actually retained? Two-thirds? Half? Maybe only ten percent? Whatever you've managed to remember, the reason you do it is due to the fact that you have somehow put it to use.

I can remember the difference between "affect" and "effect" (most of the time) because all of the writing I do has that effect. Or is it affect? Aw crap!

I can also explain to you how to format an Excel spreadsheet and write complex formulas with nested "if" statements because I do that all of the time.

Back when I taught classes on Microsoft Word and Excel, I helped my students learn by going through a series of exercises. Why? Because simply listening to me lecture on drop-down menus and dialogue boxes (aside from curing insomnia) isn't how my students learned best. Most people learn by doing. That's how ideas go from being believed (in theory) to being known (in practice).

Several years and about 60 pounds ago, I was given the opportunity to go rappelling with a group of my camping buddies. If skydiving is jumping out of a perfectly good airplane, then rappelling could be described as jumping off of a perfectly good cliff. At the time, I was a rather daring (pronounced "STOO-pid") tomboy, so despite a bit of nervousness, I was excited to give it a try.

Hiking deep into the north Georgia Mountains, we arrived at a rock outcropping on the side of a mountain with a vertical drop of about 40 feet. Our group leader, Dave, secured the rope to a tree and handed out the harnesses, which we all put on. I then watched as a few of my more experienced friends maneuvered gracefully over the side and down the cliff. Then it was my turn.

Dave turned to me and adjusted my harness so it would cut off the circulation in my legs. The rope was then secured to the harness and wound through the device that was to serve as my braking system. He patiently explained how to use the brake so that they wouldn't have to mail me back home in a bucket. Of course, it was hard to hear what he was saying over this annoying pounding in my ears, which turned out to be my heart sending me a Morse coded message, saying, "Don't do it!" However, I don't understand Morse code, so I missed the message.

Carefully, I backed up to the edge of the cliff. My brain was telling me that the rope would hold me and that my braking system would keep me from plummeting to my death. After all, I had just watched a few of the others rappel down the rock with no problems, so I had clear evidence that I wasn't in a lot of danger.

My heart, on the other hand, still wasn't buying it. Its as-yet-unheeded message changed to something akin to, "Danger, Will Robinson!" As I put more weight on the rope, my knees began to shake in syncopated rhythm with my heart's urgent warnings.

When I finally put my full weight on the rope, the nervousness vanished instantly. My heart finally understood that I wasn't going to fall. I didn't just *believe* that the rope would hold. I *knew* it would. I could *feel* it. This became my experiential Truth.

With my heart and knees satisfied, I bounded down the cliff, all the while my brain saying, "I told you so!" My brain can be a real brat sometimes.

This principle of going from believing to knowing applies to our spiritual lives as much as to our physical lives. It's one thing to believe that an idea or concept is true, especially when it is purely theoretical. It's an entirely different thing to know it so deeply that no doubt even arises. When an idea makes its way from our heads to our hearts, we gain an understanding that changes how we see ourselves and the world.

For example, I can talk all day about how judgments block our experience of Joy. I understand this concept inside out, and most of the time I live my life based around this principle.

And yet, all it takes is for a single person to push that one hot button. Suddenly I'm going on and on about how *they* need to get their act together, or how *they* have hurt me, or how what *they* are saying is a whole lot of hooey (like when I'm listening to interviews with politicians). Suddenly the Divine Law of Peace (which is what "dharmashanti" means, by the way), is totally forgotten and I am in turbocharged ego mode! Woo hoo!

Sure, I *believe* that when I judge someone, it robs me of my Peace of Mind. But obviously, I don't always *know* it.

If watching an episode of "Faze the Nation" sends me blaming the Bush administration for the price of gas, the illegal war in Iraq, and the cancellation of my favorite sitcom, there is a level on which I do not believe that judging others makes me upset. I have not completely internalized it to the point that I no longer put myself in Resentment Hell. It happens occasionally.

This is where *practicing* these principles is so essential. Every situation in our lives that triggers us is an opportunity to learn how to apply these ideas in our daily lives. As Thomas Edison said, "Genius (or spiritual mastery) is 1% inspiration and 99% perspiration." Our lives are the training grounds to work the same issues over and over and over again (fun, huh?) until Love, Compassion and Forgiveness becomes our only response.

If you've had trouble finding a completely healthy, loving, long-term relationship with someone, the relationships you've had have mostly broken up over the same basic issues. Am I right? My friend Patrick described it as having the same relationship with different faces. Been there, done that, got the tattoo!

It always baffled me why my partners would always start out so sweet, but over time would be secretly replaced by extraterrestrial pod creatures (I'm sure of it) who were emotionally unavailable, chemically addicted drama demons. Eventually, I realized the problem was me; specifically who I was attracted to and how I handled myself in the relationship. Or, as Marianne Williamson has said, "The problem isn't that you were attracted to them. The problem is that you gave them your number!"

It took me about fourteen years (plus one restraining order, two divorces, three suicide attempts, five more breakups, and roughly a dozen one-night stands with anonymous strangers...that I can remember) to recognize what was going on. All of those dysfunctional relationships (and non-relationships) were practice for learning how to Love people unconditionally, rather than trying to manipulate them. The lessons (and they are really too numerous to name here) learned from these relationships went from *what I didn't have a clue about* to *what I came to believe* and eventually to *what I now know internally.*

My relationship with my life partner of eight-plus years is unbelievable. It's like something from a fairytale. We never fight. We are able to communicate our thoughts and feelings about everything. We can even disagree without going into shaming mode or the desperate need to prove ourselves right and the other person wrong. We have maintained this level of Bliss through all kinds of challenges. This is because, in part, I don't even consider doing some of the things I used to do. I don't just *believe* the principles that make our relationship work — I *know* them.

If you want to be free from fear, you have to learn how to put your full weight on the Truth of Spiritual Principles. Practice these principles every day and give yourself permission to screw up a *lot*! You will go from believing these ideas intellectually to knowing them internally. As it says in the Bible, "You will know the Truth, and the Truth will set you free."

Chapter 13:
Conflict Happens

The Misery Conspiracy likes to complicate things that are very simple. When we are thinking negatively, we are able to come up with so many reasons why simple Love is not the best answer to a situation. Our deluded minds say, "I'd Love that person, but they did this, or that situation is an exception to the rule." When it comes to Love, there are no exceptions to the rule.

The Laws of Thermodynamics are the Laws of Thermodynamics. They don't work only some of the time. They are always true. There are no exceptions. In the same vein, the Laws of Spiritual Dynamics are also always true. If you withhold love, you feel cut off from love. There are no exceptions, not even with a note from your therapist.

Nevertheless, the Conspiracy likes to mash situations up so well, with so many twisted and intertwined threads, that we lose our sense of direction. We get so turned around that we forget the basic rules of Love.

In March 2005, it was impossible to turn on a radio or TV station without hearing about the latest court ruling or legislative action affecting the fate of Terri Schiavo. For those whose memory is as faulty as mine or who may have been visiting other planets at the time, Terri Schiavo was a severely head-injured woman in Florida who had been in a persistent vegetative state for fifteen years. Two-thirds of her brain-tissue had dissolved into liquid over the years (yeah, not a pleasant image), she had no significant brain function, and yet her heart continued to pump and she continued to breathe unaided.

The situation rose to the level of "National Media Attention" when a legal battle raged between her husband Michael, who wanted to let her die by disconnecting her feeding tube, and the Schindlers (her parents), who wanted to keep her alive by any means necessary.

Politicians, activists and pundits of all sorts selflessly (not!) threw themselves in front of oncoming television cameras, desperate for a chance to look sym-pathetic (emphasis on pathetic) to whichever side they aligned themselves with. To top it off, all three branches of national and state government (executive, legislative and judicial, in case you missed that day in Civics class) began a six-way Jell-O-wrestling match, each claiming the authority to decide the case.

Personally, I was torn between the wishes of Terri, who had previously expressed that she did not want to be kept alive by artificial means, and the agony experienced by her parents over the prolonged and impending permanent loss of their daughter. I was appalled at the willingness of both national and state governments to attempt end-runs around the court system, who had already decided the case. Similarly disheartening was the fact that the media focused only on the most superficial and divisive aspects of the situation, serving only to further polarize the issue and raise the level of hatred. Let me tell you, the Misery Conspiracy was in full force on this one!

At the core of conflict, beyond all the executive orders, legislative actions, judicial rulings, salacious news coverage and screaming protesters, was a woman caught somewhere between life and death. This was a person who had suffered brain damage, reportedly as an indirect result of an eating disorder. How ironic that the legal debate now centered on whether to feed a woman who had attempted to starve herself to death.

There was also the husband who had loved her, but who, after several devoted years of caring for his nearly brain-dead wife, felt the need to move on with his life. I am not claiming he was either a saint or a jerk. But let's face it, in such a situation, we would all get a bit lonely in what had become a one-sided relationship.

And of course, there were Terri's parents, who still desperately clung to the hope that she might one day awaken, or at least felt the need to maintain the vigil of keeping her alive physically, even if she knew nothing of their efforts. While I have never had kids of my own, I can certainly appreciate a parent's overwhelming Love for their child, especially one in need of constant care. Certainly the loss of a child is not something I could ever imagine and would not wish on anyone.

All of these people had suffered immeasurably. None of them are evil. They were just trying to make the best decisions they could. Unfortunately, these decisions were in conflict with each other. That's how life is sometimes. Just like the people who have different ideas about how to memorialize those lost in the September 11 attacks, all with the best intentions. Sometimes life just gets complicated. Conflict happens.

When I am confronted with an issue as complex as this, I am reminded that my job is really very simple. The only difficulty is remembering what my job is and what it's not. It is *not* my job to figure out who's right and who's wrong. And just in case you're wondering, that's not your job either, unless you happen to be a judge or a jury member, but that's not really what I'm talking about!

It *is* my job (and yours as well) to Love and Forgive everyone involved. It is our job to embody Compassion for all of us, to pray for Peace and healing (both physical and spiritual), especially for those we think are "in the wrong". It is our job to seek wisdom and support from the One Self. That's our job and nothing else!

Whether we have an active part to play in the situation (such as a doctor or judge or politician or family member) or are merely an observer, we have to decide what we want to contribute. At that level, we have only two choices. We can add more Love or we can add more hate.

We have to decide this before we even consider what actions to take. Too often we unconsciously turn over that responsibility to our negative thought process, which inevitably chooses to crank up the hate, judgment and misery. What else would it choose? It is a thought process programmed by the Misery Conspiracy! Our consciousness is asleep at the wheel. God may be our co-pilot, but most of the time it's the Misery Conspiracy that's steering the plane. It's time we wake up and consciously choose Love if we ever want to experience Peace and Joy.

That means we have to start with Love, not with the details of the situation. Looking at the Schiavo case as the media presented it, we see only heartbreak, hatred, fear, and a lot of cheap drama. However, if we start with loving everyone involved, we rise above all of the garbage and are drawn to helping everyone find Peace.

When all we want is to extend Love to the people involved, we are naturally drawn to the most enlightened approach to the so-called crisis. Once we make that choice, Love instinctively manifests itself without our conscious effort. We plug into the One Self and become conduits for creating Heaven on Earth. That is what the Peace Prayer of St. Francis is all about. Maybe that seems all "unicorns and rainbows" to you (hey, I like rainbows, so BACK OFF!), but it is truly the most practical approach to any situation.

Wherever Terri Schiavo is, I send her loving, healing energy with wishes for Joy in the next stage of her journey (she's not dead, she just moved on and left us squabbling at each other). I ask for emotional healing for both her husband and her family. They have all suffered so much through all of this. There are no villains, only people who need Love and Compassion. I pray also for all of the politicians and lobbyists and healthcare workers, that they may find the most loving direction in their journeys.

Birth is not a beginning. Death is not an end. They are both just stages of our journey to learn how to remove the blocks to our awareness of Love. Apparently everybody forgot this during Terri's last days. By design, our spiritual journeys draw us into situations that demand we break down our barriers to Love.

When we find ourselves dealing with, or at least thinking about, a complex situation, we simply have to break it down to the level of content. Don't let the thinking of the Misery Conspiracy, with all of its emphasis on exceptions, distract you.

Focus on what the Laws of Spiritual Dynamics tell us. Will we respond with Compassion or judgment? Do we want to get lost in the drama or would we rather experience inner Peace? Choose Love and you will experience Peace. Choose to withhold it and, the ego will steer your little plane right into a building.

Chapter 14:
How Sad

A critical lesson for anyone who wants to defeat the Misery Conspiracy is learning how to change perspectives. As bright and open-minded as we may be, all of us have serious blind spots. We have a tendency to overlook some things that we would rather not deal with right now. This may include certain behaviors or attitudes that we consciously or subconsciously keep tucked away.

No matter what age we happened to be, there is this unspoken sense that we are as smart as we are going to get. I used to keep a personal journal to help me deal with some of the issues that I was going through. Years later, I made the mistake of actually reading what I wrote. I cringed. What was I thinking? To this day, I have trouble keeping my blog (an online journal) going for more than a couple of weeks. I keep getting flashbacks to that drivel I wrote years ago.

When I was a teenager, I actually wrote a collection of essays and it was almost published. I signed a book deal and everything. By the grace of God (at least for my sake, not theirs), the publisher went out of business shortly after I sent back the edited galleys. When I stumbled on a copy of the manuscript years later (I think I was in the process of moving), I started reading some of it. Some of the essays were quite insightful for a teenager. Others made me wonder who this person was to have blindly accepted certain concepts or to have drawn such naïve conclusions. Nevertheless, it made a good fireplace starter that winter.

Over the years, I have practiced a long series of different religious traditions (Catholicism, Charismatic Christianity, Wicca, Buddhism, etc.). As I worked through some of my personal issues, including addiction, codependency and depression, and accepted certain aspects of who I am (such as my gender identity and sexual orientation), I have been drawn to different spiritual paths. Or maybe it's just different sections of the same path, who knows? Either way, my perspective has evolved.

Shortly before I came to terms with being transgender, I was living in midtown Atlanta and was a member of a very conservative, very prominent church, not far from my home. One June morning, I was driving home after services. I found myself waiting at a stoplight that was holding red to allow the gay pride parade to pass by. I sat in my car, shaking my head and thinking to myself, "How sad!" I felt that the people in that parade had been drawn into a sinful lifestyle and that they risked going to Hell if they didn't repent. That's what I had been taught. And like the rest of us, I didn't know any better.

Of course, a lot can happen in a year, and in my case *a whole lot* happened by the next June. I came out of the closet, began living life as a woman, and was finally at Peace with myself. The doctrines of hate and judgment had been tossed in my mental dumpster. I had lost much of what made up my old life, including my home, my marriage, my family, and my job. I had been since kicked out of my church. They apparently had a hard time allowing a person like me to worship God.

A year after the day I had watched that parade go by my church, I was in the parade. And as we passed by my old church, I saw members of the church holding signs that said "God hates fags" and "Matthew Shepherd burns in hell", among other horribly, un-Christ-like rhetoric.

I recognized a few of the people holding the signs. I remembered that day a year ago, when I was passing judgment on the people in the parade. I looked at the people with the hateful signs, shook my head and said to myself, "How sad."

This time, I wasn't thinking that the people I was looking at were bad or evil. I just realized that they had been brainwashed with fear and flawed theology. It even occurred to me that it was possible that one of those people holding the signs may be struggling with their sexuality or gender. My hope was that one day, they too would know Peace. I prayed that they would eventually be able to let go of their hate and discover the unconditional love that Jesus shared.

It is said that we should not judge another person until we have walked a mile in their shoes. And I have also heard some add, "So that when they get mad at you for proving them wrong, they will be a mile away and barefoot."

We need to be open to new points of view and allow our perspective to continuously evolve as we experience new situations and meet new people. We have to allow for the possibility that the way we see things now may be based on assumptions, judgments and agendas. We could be dead wrong in some of our beliefs, and that ideas we cherish today may make us cringe five or ten years from now. We may look back and say, "How sad!"

Chapter 15:
The Ugly Road to Acceptance

One of my biggest challenges is accepting things as they are. This includes accepting other people as they are, without feeling the compulsion to control them or worse, fix them. This challenge of acceptance includes my refusal to accept certain aspects of who I am. The consequence of this lack of acceptance was a collection of addictive and compulsive behaviors that, for years, robbed me of my Peace of mind and frequently put me in precarious situations. To this day, it amazes me that I am still alive after some of the things I've done.

I struggled for a long time with my issues of gender. It wasn't my plan to be "different". I always preferred to blend in with everyone else, to be one of the crowd. But I have known from an early age that I was not "normal" (whatever *that* is). As I became an adult, it became ever clearer that I was transgender.

Having grown up in the 70's and 80's, I had seen how gay and transgender people were portrayed and treated. I didn't want that. I wanted to be a good little Christian, go to Church twice a week, and have a successful career with a happy family of 2.7 children.

I went to therapy and counseling to help me with my "condition". I prayed. I read my Bible. I participated in the music team at church. And if that wasn't enough, I overcompensated by going to bars and sleeping with strange men; a compulsive behavior that I found myself powerless to stop. Every time I did it, I spent hours afterward bawling my eyes out, praying for God to make me stop. But the insanity continued.

Then one day, I picked up three guys at once at one of the bars. We drove to one of their houses for another round of anonymous sex. But at the last minute decided I didn't want to sleep with them. They apparently weren't concerned with what I wanted and spent the next half hour gang-raping me. I cried for days after that.

I realized that it was time to accept myself for who I was. I was different. I was being lead down a different road than the one that I had been told was mine. And with this acceptance, I found Peace. The compulsive behaviors and insane, obsessive thought processes vanished. I saw that I could begin a new life.

Mind you, I still had a lot of lessons to learn. A few years into my new life, I met Ray. We started out as friends, but quickly fell in love with each other. I began to think that I could go back to a normal life. But what I didn't realize was that we were both ticking time bombs. While my compulsive drinking and other behaviors had diminished, I still harbored some negative self-perceptions that began to manifest into codependency.

Ray had issues of his own. He was dealing with issues of low self-esteem as well, but his manifested into emotional coldness and rage. As the newness of our relationship began to fade, our inner demons began to surface and we became like fire and gas. I manipulated and tried to coerce him into loving me. He screamed and belittled and interrogated.

What was my solution to this? What else? I decided that we should get married. Notice that I said, "I decided". He wasn't keen on the idea. But being the master manipulator I was, I was determined to get him to marry me, because of course, everyone knows that getting married can make a bad relationship better. Imagine my surprise when things got worse!

Now on top of his existing issues with me, Ray resented me for coercing him into getting married. He raged at me even more, and I begged and pleaded and cried and whined that much more. He would go off to bars and sleep around on me, while I wailed at home and contemplated suicide. What a lovely picture of the American dream we were.

When we both lost our jobs one week in December, *I decided* that this would be our chance to make a new start and move to a new city 2200 miles (AA calls this a "geographic"). Again, please note that I said, "I decided". It took a week of talking and encouraging and spinning and selling before he was willing to consider moving from Atlanta to Phoenix. Part of his reluctance stemmed from the fact that moving meant leaving his young daughter behind with his ex-wife. But I was the master of manipulation and by New Years Eve, we were moved into our new apartment in the Valley of the Sun.

Now Ray resented me for pushing him to abandon his daughter in addition to getting married. We both added out-of-control drinking to our repertoires of insanity, as our marriage when from dysfunctional to destructive. I started hanging out at the local lesbian bars and getting smashed. Then I'd call Ray to pick me up because I was too drunk to drive. I don't know which was worse: my husband finding out I was gay or my lesbian friends finding out I was married. Either way, I felt humiliated.

Eventually, I attempted suicide and again found myself at the bottom emotionally and spiritually. And again, I realized that part of what I need was acceptance; not from anyone else, but from myself.

I had to accept that I had a drinking problem. I had to accept that I had some serious codependency problems. I had to accept that while I cared very deeply for Ray, we both had a lot of issues that made a romantic relationship between us impossible. And when I accepted all of this, I was finally able to deal with the issues and get on with my life...AGAIN. Denying the truth and resisting the need to deal with the problems made the problems worse. Accepting them provided me the starting point to deal with them.

It is important that we get an honest assessment of our current situation, especially if we want to change it. In the 12-Step process, we call this taking a personal inventory. We recognize the dynamics of what's going on. We pay particular attention to what we are doing that contributes to the situation being what it is. We don't focus on blame or guilt. Rather, we look to see how our attitudes and actions have made the situation worse, and then consider how we can change ourselves.

In the case of my marriage to Ray, I had to see that my attitudes towards myself and towards him were keeping me stuck in an unhealthy relationship. By accepting that I had some responsibility for my being where I was, I could then accept responsibility for getting out by changing the decisions that I had been making. I could stop drinking. I could go to meetings to share my experiences and get support. I could pray and meditate and read 12-Step literature. I could let go of my need for Ray's approval. I could decide to take care of my needs, including the need to live in a safe and sane environment. And that's what I did.

I also accepted that Ray was where he was. I accepted that he was an alcoholic, just like me. I accepted that while there was a lot I could do about my own disease, there was nothing I could do for him. I was not in control of him. I was not in control of his drinking or his raging or his infidelities. When I accepted that, it took off a lot of the pressure that I had put myself under. In a sense, I surrendered to the reality of the situation. And in doing so, I could change it.

I am constantly accepting new things about myself. I have had to accept that as I've gotten older, my memory isn't what it used to be. And in accepting that, I have learned to develop processes so that I know where I need to be. I have accepted that my housekeeping skills aren't the best in the world. In fact, my decorating style isn't modern or contemporary or even late Victorian. It's more early college. And that's okay. As long as my spouse Eileen can live with it, so can I.

If you are in a situation that is making you crazy, start by accepting the situation for what it is. If you are dealing with clinical depression, admit it and accept it. If you are addicted to alcohol, drugs or anything else, accept it. If you have an unhealthy relationship with a significant other or a family member or even your boss, accept the other person for who they are and let go of any expectations that they are going to change any time soon. And accept your part for making the relationship the way it is.

Accepting things as they are doesn't mean you give up hope of improving things. It simply means that you are getting an accurate measurement of what is going on. From there you can make conscious changes to your own thoughts and actions. You don't try to change anyone else. You just do what you need to do to take care of yourself.

If you've been dishonest about anything, you start being rigorously honest with yourself and those around you. If you've been judgmental, you let go of your judgments. If you've been letting people walk all over you, then you learn to set and honor your boundaries.

Just as the first step in recovering from addiction is accepting that we have a problem, the first step in dealing with whatever struggles *you* face is accepting them as they are. From there you will be equipped to make the best decisions to create a future that is different from the past.

Chapter 16:
Welcome to the Garden

There is a place I go every week where I can be totally real. It is a beautiful place full of rich colors, amazing artwork, tantalizing foods, sensuous aromas and the most amazing people in the world. In this place, people gather to laugh, to cry, to share their incredible stories, to read inspirational writings and to help each other grow in their spiritual journey.

This place is not a church or a mosque or a temple of any kind. It is simply an informal gathering that we call the Garden Club (not to be confused with the Garden Club of America). Started by my mentor Kaay in 1994, it is open to every woman that feels the call to join. There are no dues or attendance requirements. We simply gather, eat and enjoy the blessing of each other's company.

Describing Garden Club is like trying to describe the experience of eating mango for the first time. Even words like sweet, juicy, and tingly are no substitute for that first cold bite of mango. Likewise, nothing I say here can truly convey the miraculous weekly experience that is my Garden Club women's circle. And yet I would be remiss in my duties if I did not try.

These women are sisters and mothers and aunts and daughters and grandmothers to each other. We have had women from India and Israel, Germany and Russia, Morocco and Nigeria, Costa Rica and Vietnam. We are black and brown and white, Jewish and Christian and Muslim and Sikh and atheist, straight and gay and transgender. We have had women as young as 12 and older than 80. We have helped each other through the deaths of loved ones (including a few members), divorces, illnesses, births, and bankruptcies. Some of us are addicted to alcohol, drugs, dysfunctional relationships and food, while others have never been addicted to anything.

Another dynamic that makes Garden Club such a safe place is the non-judgment. There is no finger-pointing and very little advice giving. Rather we share our struggles in an open, trusting space, and allow others to relate similar experiences and how they worked through them. Our goal is to help each other become the best that she can be.

The result of this magnificent group is that the women who come, many of whom have been traumatized in one way or many, go from being victims to survivors to glorious goddesses. Had it not been for Garden Club, dozens and perhaps hundreds of women may have ended up on the streets, in jail or dead, often dragging their families with them. Garden Club is saving the world in ways that no government agency could and that few religious institutions know how.

I share this with you because there is no reason why this magical, healing experience should belong to the women of Garden Club alone. We hold in our circle the secret to transforming the world. It is a secret that must be shared if we are to survive as a planet.

If you don't already belong to a group like this, start one! Yes, you! When my mentor Kaay started Garden Club more than a decade ago, the idea of bringing a bunch of women into her home every week terrified her. She didn't like women. She didn't trust women. But it was what she felt called to do. Many years later, she cherishes the women that have found their way to the circle and to her life.

When we started out, there wasn't the free flow of loving conversation that we have now. We began by taking turns reading out of Sherry Anderson's book, *The Feminine Face of God*. We'd read a little and then we'd talk about it. And we'd read a little more and we'd talk about that. Then we moved on to other books such as

Julia Cameron's *The Artist's Way* and Clarissa Pinkola Estés' *Women Who Run with the Wolves.*

The women of the circle began to come out of their shells and remove their masks. We allowed ourselves to be completely honest and real with each other. Deep spiritual connections began to form creating a chain of compassion, love and support that has lasted over the years and has extended out into the world. It is more powerful than words can describe.

If you feel a stirring to create such a group, I encourage you to go for it. Trust the process. Reach out to people, particularly those who are different from you. The women of Garden Club have found great strength in their diversity. When I first joined, I was this young, tough trans-dyke with less than a year of sobriety. I soon met a woman by the name of Linda, who grew up in a tiny town in North Dakota; very prim and proper. Nothing like me!

When I was introduced to her, I thought to myself, "Well, she seems nice, but I have *nothing* to learn from her "Prairie Home Companion" ways." Boy was I wrong! I have learned to love this woman and respect her for all that she brings to life and to the circle. She is awesome! But I had to allow for her difference in order to learn what she had to teach.

If you're thinking of starting a spiritual circle, let me suggest some ground rules. First, no alcohol or mood-altering drugs. One of the things that makes these spiritual circles so powerful is the ability for everyone to be themselves. Alcohol and drugs interfere with that process of honesty and trust.

Also if you are going to be a gender-specific group, don't spend your time bashing the other gender. Garden Club is limited to women, but we are by no means a "man-hater's" club. While we prefer to maintain the boundary of womanhood in the circle, we honor the masculine as well as the feminine in us and in the men in our lives.

Try opening your circle with a simple, non-religious prayer, allowing anyone with needs to offer up their special concerns and prayers for themselves or others. We call it putting someone or something (including cars, refrigerators and the odd laptop) into the circle.

What you do from there is up to you. Just create a space where it is safe for everyone to share and laugh and cry and celebrate and commiserate and, most of all, grow. Oh, and keep lots of tissues handy.

At Garden Club, we don't plant flowers or trees or herbs. We are about growing ourselves. We are about sharing our wisdom, both ancient and new, from all of our diverse traditions. This is the light towards which we all grow.

Chapter 17:
Wag the Drunk

One of the biggest lessons we can take from the wonderful world of medicine is the necessity to treat diseases and not just their symptoms. Treating the symptoms may provide temporary relief, but it allows the disease to go underground. When it re-emerges at a later time, perhaps in a new form, it is often much stronger than before.

In 2005, the Food & Drug Administration approved a drug that is supposed to help alcoholics overcome their cravings for alcohol. (I'm still waiting for the drug that will help me overcome my craving for coffee and books.) While non-alcoholics may view this breakthrough as quite an accomplishment, most of us who have struggled with the diseases of addiction know that no drug by itself can cure us.

Alcoholism isn't a drinking problem. It's a stopping problem. Before I got sober, I was *really good* at drinking. But stopping after one or two drinks was a different story. It's not that I craved the alcohol per se; well, at least not ALL of the time. (No, that's not denial. No, really it's not! It's not! Oh, STOP it!) It's just that a whole lot of drinks provided a brief vacation from my overwhelming feelings of worthlessness and despair. I was engaging in insane behavior to stop my insane thinking. That's all any addiction is, whether the drug of choice is alcohol, meth or reality TV.

Even when I did manage to stop drinking, my life continued to whirl out of control. I still found myself attracted to people who were emotionally unavailable or abusive. I still had suicidal thoughts. I still had no clue how to handle all of the crazy dramas going on in my life. My life was like a non-stop movie fest on the Lifetime Network. The booze was gone, but I was still struggling with what my mentor Kaay calls "the fumes."

Early on in my recovering, I would go to AA and Al-Anon meetings and ask people if I should abandon my abusive marriage or try to stick it out. Every time I asked, I got the same response, "Just wait. The answer will come to you."

That drove me crazy (like I needed more "crazy"). I was desperate for a solution to this issue, and these people were refusing to give it to me. I was convinced that they really *did* know, but didn't want to let me in on the secret. Can we say "paranoid"? Again, no alcohol, but the insanity continued. The fumes, you see...

As it turns out, the real reason why I couldn't get an answer for my marriage situation was because it took time for me to work through my "stinkin' thinkin'." Even if someone had told me to leave my husband (which I eventually did), I would have fallen in love with the next head case I found remotely attractive. (Oh, wait a minute, I did that, too. Her name was Debbie.) In order to break the cycle, I had to approach the situation from a totally different direction. I had to learn to open my mind to thinking based on Love rather than fear. I had to hear a new voice.

An addiction is our negative thought process at full-turbo overdrive with nitro boosters! It is the Misery Conspiracy's *pièce de resistance*. As addicts, our minds are totally consumed with loveless, selfish thoughts about *everything*! Any other way of thinking is incomprehensible...and well, boring. For an addict caught in the monster's belly, there is no light, no hope and no Love.

Most addicts I know are multiply addicted. It's our form of multi-tasking. I was addicted not only to alcohol, but also to emotionally unavailable people, anonymous sex, tobacco, food, suicidal thoughts, and probably a few others that I have forgotten. We addicts are willing to try just about anything to avoid dealing with our real issues.

So a drug that curbs an alcoholic's craving for booze may ease things a little, but it's not going to "cure" the disease any more than an anesthetic cures a gunshot wound. It may ease the pain, and may even help us stay sober long enough to make some progress. It won't fix the real problem, however. Unless the issues of fear, denial, and isolation are addressed, addicts always relapse. Simply treating the manifestations of our disease of insanity is just wagging the drunk!

What's wagging the drunk? It's backward logic, a reference to the tail wagging the dog. It's the belief that treating the symptoms of drinking or craving alcohol will cure the disease of addiction. It's insane thinking, and believe me, we don't need any help in *that* department.

It comes down to this. If you have a problem, you have to deal with it at the level of cause rather than effect. The cause in this case isn't the decision to take a drink. It's all of the negative thoughts and beliefs and emotions that lead one to believe that drinking oneself into oblivion is a good idea.

To deal with the cause, we must confront all of the yucky (it's a technical term) thoughts and beliefs and emotions that are making us miserable. We've gotta clean out the old mental septic tank. Fun, huh? But if we really want to be rid of the addictions and not just wag the drunk, that's what we have to do.

Chapter 18:
Go Away! Can't You See I'm Meditating?!

As I mentioned before, lessons often come disguised as something else. We think we should be doing one thing, and suddenly life sends us in another direction. What's really funny is when we ask for guidance, and then don't recognize it when it comes. Be careful what you wish for — you will get it. This includes results we get from our regular spiritual practices.

Meditation is a part of my daily ritual. It's my way of undoing the damage the Misery Conspiracy continuously inflicts on my psyche. Unlike some spiritual practitioners, I'm not one of those morning people who meditate as soon as she wakes up. In fact, I am usually well into my day before I actually take the time to do it.

So for those of you who still have trouble fitting meditation into your morning routine, don't beat up on yourself too much. You're in good company. And to those "Type A" people who do it before their feet hit the floor, I say, "Must be nice."

But, this chapter isn't about when we meditate. It's about what happens when we open ourselves to the process...the Big Process...the Universal, Divine Process.

When I was working as a temp for the City of Phoenix, I often meditated during my mid-morning break inside City Hall's cathedralesque atrium. It was a chance to get my meditation time in, and, of course, to give any passersby something to wonder about. (Is she asleep? Is she alive? Hit it with a rock!)

Once I made the mistake (or was it?) of choosing a somewhat high-traffic spot, just outside my work area. Having meditated for many years now, foot traffic doesn't distract me much. I can meditate on a lurching bus and in a bustling café.

On this morning, I closed my eyes and started my meditation by saying, "God, show me what you want me to do. Show me where you want me to go. Tell me what you want me to say." Then I let my mind go silent, listening to the Voice of the One Self, and allowing it to guide my mind to where I needed to be spiritually.

Most of the time when I do this, I am guided to let go of my judgments and to simply be at Peace. The response I got this time, however, seemed more like a distraction than guidance. Only a few moments after I had expressed my openness to God, my friend Evelyn walked by and asked, "How can you possibly meditate here?"

I opened my eyes. "Practice. Lots of practice," I said with a smile. What I really wanted to say was, "Go away! Can't you see I'm meditating?"

I do enjoy talking with Evelyn, but at the moment I really wanted to do some "serious" spiritual work. Then she opened up about some problems she'd been having with her mother. Listening to someone complain about their family was not how I wanted to spend my meditation time. Nevertheless, I listened (impatiently) and then shared with her a few insights about her situation. By that time, my break was over. My chance to meditate had indeed been lost. What a waste!

But it wasn't really a waste. It occurred to me that helping Evelyn was perhaps what God *wanted me to do*. That spot was precisely where I was supposed to be. The insights that suddenly popped into my head during our conversation were exactly *what needed to be said*. I realized that during what little meditating I did, I had asked for the opportunity to serve the Universal Good; to be open to the process. That's what I got. Be careful what you ask for.

The goal of meditation is to connect to the Divine and to become available to the process of undoing all of the loveless thinking in the world. It is the process of becoming an instrument of Peace. But it's not enough to be open to the process in theory. We must take an active part. That was my lesson when Evelyn interrupted my meditation. When you say, "Use me" to the One Self, don't get all bent out of shape when the response is, "Okay, do this!"

My mentor Kaay, is always saying, "Trust the process." This is crucial advice! We have this tendency to freak out when the Universe isn't showing us what we want. When this happens to me, I either shut myself off from the process or try to control it. Neither is very productive and both show a lack of understanding of how things work.

Instead, we must make ourselves available to our own healing process. Be willing to show up when someone has a need. Try not to let unexpected turns throw you. Be willing to see things differently. As we begin to trust the Universal Process, what shows up in our life and how we experience it will dramatically change for the better!

Chapter 19:
Never Lost

Not only do situations have the opportunity to teach us how to get ourselves out from under the grip of the Misery Conspiracy; technology can have the same effect. Now, I'm not a technical whiz; at least not compared to my partner, Eileen. She is amazing when it comes to all things mechanical and electronic. And like most techies, she loves gadgets!

A few years ago, Eileen and I flew out to California to spend some time with a cousin. At the Oakland airport, we rented a car with a Hertz Neverlost® GPS navigation system. For Eileen, it was love at first bleep. And I have to confess, I was impressed, too. This ingenious device allowed us to enter the address of a destination (e.g. her cousin's house) and it would verbally guide us turn by turn until we arrived.

As if that weren't remarkable enough, if we failed to turn where instructed, the Neverlost® would tell us that we missed a turn and would then re-calculate directions from our current location. Amazing technology, except of course for those guys who prefer to wander around until they figure it out for themselves, or run out of gas in the middle of nowhere!

So how does this relate to spirituality? Well, every situation we encounter in our daily lives has the potential to teach us something important. In most cases, it's that crucial lesson that would make our lives a whole lot easier if we'd only get it. Through

Divine Design and the use of state-of-the-art Cosmic Technology, our lives are customized for maximum enlightenment training.

Our Internal Teacher, what some call the One Self or Intuition or the Holy Spirit, is comparable to a spiritual Neverlost® system. When we listen to the gentle, loving directions of that Sacred Inner Voice, we learn the lessons we need to learn quickly, easily, and relatively painlessly.

However, when we fail to learn from a situation (i.e., miss a turn), the One Self says, "Okay, you missed that lesson. That's okay. Let me make some adjustments to your divine directions. It will take a little longer, but you will get there." Then we somehow find ourselves re-routed and facing a similar situation with the same lessons to learn.

My friend, Jayda, learned this lesson the hard way, as we all do sometimes. Jayda had been self-employed back in the early 1990s and had found herself owing nearly $50,000 in income taxes. For years she did everything to avoid dealing with it because the amount was overwhelming. There was no way she could pay those taxes.

She was forced onto a payroll deduction plan, then managed to get out of it when she became self-employed again. Nevertheless, the IRS haunted Jayda. She started to make an Offer in Compromise, but withdrew it when the attorney told her that there was a good chance that the IRS would reject it, leaving her owing an attorney's bill on top of the taxes, penalties and interest.

Years later, she filed for bankruptcy, thinking *finally* she had slipped out of the IRS' icy grip. But to no avail. As it turned out, her home had increased in value enough to attract the IRS' attention. They threatened to take her house. Finally, she was willing to face her debt, refinanced her home, and paid the taxes.

My point here isn't to tell you to pay your taxes or else. Rather, it's a classic example of a problem creeping up over and over until you finally do what you need to do and learn the lessons to be learned.

In this case, the lesson for Jayda was to face her fears and not ignore her problems. I've done the same things in relationships, going through one painful breakup after another before finally realizing that there was something about me that was causing the situation to repeat itself.

Our Internal Teacher doesn't make us feel guilty for missing a lesson. Any guilt we experience comes from that other voice; the one that speaks for the Misery Conspiracy. Our Internal Teacher, on the other hand, gently and lovingly reminds us to open ourselves up to the process, to let go of judgments, and to be willing to see things differently. We then get rerouted to resume our journey towards enlightenment.

The next time you lose your cool with someone, you've missed an opportunity to let go of fear. But it's no big deal. Just re-focus on what your Internal Teacher is telling you and get it the next time. Or the time after that. It's not important how many wrong turns we make or even the extent to which our own loveless thinking steers us off course. Eventually, we will all make it Home.

Chapter 20:
Parable of the Pagan Lesbian

Sometimes an old story just needs to be refreshed with more modern symbols in order for us to really get the lesson. Cultural and historical symbols don't always translate into another society or time. The Chevy Nova was never a big hit in Mexico because "no va," in Spanish literally means "it doesn't go". And when Coca-Cola's slogan "Coke adds life" was used in Japan, it got (mis)translated as "Coke brings your ancestors back from the dead." The Japanese were not happy!

In that spirit, the following is a modern (and might I add, *true*) re-telling of Jesus' parable of the Good Samaritan. I share this because we find it difficult for some reason to really apply the symbolic meaning of the parable into the modern context of our lives.

At the time that Jesus told this parable, a few of his critics were playing "Stump the Radical Rabbi" with him. One of his interrogators asked him to name the greatest commandment of all time. A tricky question, to be sure. But Jesus was up to the task. He replied, "Love God unconditionally. And the second greatest is similar. Love your neighbor unconditionally as you Love yourself unconditionally." Ding! Ding! Ding! Jesus scores 100 points!

But that's not the end of the story. Jesus' answer naturally prompted the next question, "Who is my neighbor?" At this point, Jesus decided to give his listeners a reality check. Everyone was expecting something like, "Love your fellow Jews." But Jesus knew it was time people broadened their worldview a bit. Rather than give a simplistic answer, he chose instead to use a parable with an unlikely protagonist: a Samaritan.

As you may know, in those days Samaritans were considered to be bad news! Unclean! Evil! They were the Palestinians (at least in the eyes of Jews) of their day. Everyone had been taught from birth that God was going to send the Samaritans to Hell! So for Jesus to make a Samaritan the hero of his story was enough to put the word "blasphemer" on the lips of his listeners. But perhaps it also made them reconsider the way they had viewed outsiders.

And who are the Samaritans of today? Okay, aside from Palestinians. Who is it that the religious and political authorities are constantly railing about and condemning? How about gays, transsexuals, Muslims, homeless people, and undocumented aliens?

We still forget that "Love your neighbor unconditionally" applies to the Samaritans of our day. That was precisely Jesus' point. We need to Love *all* people unconditionally, not just those who are like us or whom we are told to like by the Misery Conspiracy. Sometimes the ones that we have dismissed and condemned to Hell are the ones that we may depend on later. Thus begins *my* version of the story:

~~~~~~~~~~~~~~~~~~~~~~~~~~~~

In the city of Tucson lived a woman named Martha. She was a good, churchgoing woman. But as fate would have it, she began to suffer from serious health problems. By the time her doctors determined the nature of her illness, her kidneys had failed, forcing her to undergo dialysis every other day. She lost her job and found herself on welfare, struggling to survive physically and financially.

She asked her sister to donate one of her kidneys to her. But her sister refused for fear that she, too, might contract the same illness and would need a kidney from someone else. So Martha turned to the support of her fellow church members.

Every week for months, her request was put forth to the congregation for anyone with type O+ blood, the most common
~~~~~~~~~~~~~~~~~~~~~~~~~~~~

blood type, to consider being tested as a possible kidney donor. But week after week, no one came forward; not even to be tested as a match.

Finally, after several months of painful dialysis, Martha once more asked the congregation for help. As it happened, two visitors were in attendance that Sunday. The visitors were Della, a former member who now lived 100 miles away, and her lesbian partner, Shannon. Shannon was not a Christian. She was a pagan, worshipping both God and Goddess. The couple was in town to pick up a few things that had been left in a storage locker.

When Shannon heard the request she felt led to respond. When the church service was over, Shannon answered Martha's desperate call for help by agreeing to be tested as a donor. Shannon knew nothing about Martha or about what was involved with donating a kidney. She was just willing to help. She was available to the greater Process.

For nine months, Shannon endured test after test to make sure that she was the ideal candidate for the transplant. She encountered resistance from the transplant team because only once before in America had a stranger donated a kidney, and never in Arizona.

"Why would you want to do such a thing?" they asked her.

"Because she needs it. What else would I do?" she replied.

During this period of medical and psychological testing, Martha lost her apartment. The transplant team took her off the recipient list because she was no longer in a position to maintain a kidney if she received one. When Shannon and Della heard about this, they went out and paid for a new apartment for Martha to live in until she could return to a normal life and support herself. Martha was overwhelmed.

Finally, Shannon was approved to be a donor to Martha. The transplant took place and within a few months, Martha was once again supporting herself with a new job. She no longer had to suffer the agony of dialysis. She had been given a new chance in life with a precious gift, not from a relative or a fellow Christian, but by a woman that some would have condemned to Hell.

~~~~~~~~~~~~~~~~~~~~~~~~~~~~

As I said before, the above parable is a true story. The names have been changed to honor the anonymity of the people involved. There were no news reports of the transplant; no appearances on Oprah, no interviews on NPR. It wasn't about fame or celebrity status. It was about people being available to help each other, even if they were strangers and even if society in general had rejected them as unworthy of Love.

Who is your neighbor? Your neighbors are the gays and the undocumented immigrants and the pagans and the transsexuals. They are the terrorists and the hate-mongering talk show hosts and the corrupt politicians and the dishonest lobbyists. They are the abused children and the homeless people. Your neighbors are everyone you come in contact with or think about.

You are called to Love every one of your neighbors unconditionally, to be there for them and to support them, just as you do for yourself. It is our lovelessness that blocks the Joy of Heaven from our experience. It is hate and judgment that keeps us trapped in the Misery Conspiracy. And it is Love that will lift us above the insanity and bring us to our natural state of Divine Peace. Love your neighbor with all your heart—or if need be, with all your kidney!
~~~~~~~~~~~~~~~~~~~~~~~~~~~~

Chapter 21:
The Cosmic Karmic Council

As I explained in the previous chapter, cultural differences often cause us to miss the meaning of certain borrowed concepts. The Yiddish phrase, *Mazel tov,* is a great example of this. Often it is used by Jews and non-Jews alike to wish someone congratulations. Literally, however, it means "good luck." I find that rather appropriate, especially when it's said at weddings. *Oh, you just got married? Well, good luck with THAT!*

Another concept lost in cultural translation is *karma,* which comes from the spiritual traditions of India and Asia. Because Eastern and Western religions are so strikingly different, our understanding of karma has been skewed. We took the idea of karma and twisted it into the paranoia and guilt that makes Western culture the glorious icon that it isn't. To illustrate how such a wonderful thing as karma can get so warped, let me share a story about my friend Denise.

Denise has had more drama in her life than the worst soap opera. She never graduated high school because her family forced her to work a full time job since she was fifteen. Her mother and stepfather kicked her out of the house on her eighteenth birthday. By the age of 26, she had three kids, each with a different father who was either in prison, on drugs, or violent.

Denise suspected that her current boyfriend (not the father of any of her kids) was having more than a casual relationship with her best friend. This "friend" would frequently stop by during the day when the boyfriend was babysitting the kids, while Denise struggled to support the entire family on her miniscule income.

In Denise's favor, she really loved her kids and made a valiant effort at loving her boyfriend. She worked hard at her job, but she couldn't get promoted for lack of a diploma or a G.E.D. It seemed that the Universe had really dealt her a bad hand. Once she asked me if I thought she had bad karma. Maybe, I thought.

I hear a lot of talk about karma — particularly "bad karma." If something bad happens to us, we want to blame it on bad karma, as if it were some kind of divine punishment for our mistakes. *We blow a tire. It must be karma. It rains on our vacation. It must be karma. The dog poops on our brand new $500 bedspread. It must be karma.*

It's as if the Cosmic Karmic Council of the Misery Conspiracy (comprised of God, Buddha, and Santa Claus) is keeping track of all of the stupid stuff we've done in our lives and is just waiting for the chance to bring the world crashing down on our heads! *Oooh, scary! Better be good or Karma's gonna getcha!!!* I've got news for you, folks! It doesn't work that way!

Karma has nothing to do with our past. Really! Absolutely nothing! To think that the Divine Mind of God, the Consciousness of Love, would wish us anything but Joy is ridiculous. A lot of people think God is angry at them for making mistakes. So when something unpleasant or unexpected happens, they think that God or Karma is punishing them. Nothing could be further from the truth.

Karma is all about the present moment and it's all about us. Specifically, it's about how we see ourselves. *Are we loveable or not loveable? Are we guilty or are we innocent? Do we deserve to be happy or do we deserve to be miserable? Are we willing to nurture ourselves or sabotage ourselves?* These attitudes and self-perceptions are where karma comes from. Not from anything in the past.

I have heard some spiritual teachers say that when we engage in a loveless act, it takes years and sometimes millennia to burn off the negative karma. Yeah, whatever! If we ignore the lessons the Universe is sending our way and continue to see ourselves as unworthy, it may indeed take thousands of years to let go of our guilt, resentments, and other loveless thoughts.

The disasters and disappointments that we attribute to negative karma is nothing more than the result of our negative thinking. Rather than take responsibility for our own attitudes and actions, we find it a lot easier to blame our misfortunes on some mysterious principle called "Bad Karma".

For a better understanding of the way karma *really* works, let's take another look at my friend Denise. She got kicked out of the house on her eighteenth birthday. Now I will be the first to admit that that's not how I would want to spend my birthday. But was it a bad thing or a good thing?

Sometimes stuff just happens. Life with her stepfather wasn't exactly pleasant to begin with. According to Denise, he seemed to have problems keeping his hands and other parts of his anatomy off his step-daughters. Alcoholism or other addictions were rampant in the home as well. Could it be that her getting kicked out was a chance to get away from all of that? What if "the Cosmic Karmic Council" wasn't trying to punish her? What if it was trying to get her away from that dysfunctional household? Is it scary to be on one's own at eighteen? Of course, it is. But perhaps the road to recovery led right out that front door!

Then there are Denise's relationship issues. Oh, boy! What are the odds of falling in Love with one deadbeat psycho after another? They all seemed so nice at first, but then something always happened to change them. Imagine that!

As someone who has had more than her share of nightmare relationships, I can definitely speak to that. When we find ourselves picking one loser after another, the problem doesn't lie entirely with the other person. Clearly our "picker" is broken, because out of the hundreds of people we come in contact with, we keep picking these gems!

It's easy to blame karma for your run of bad relationships, but if you're the one picking these people out of a crowd, you're "picker" is broken. I know mine was. My partner of eight plus years is not the kind of person I would normally be attracted to (not enough drama going on), which is precisely why our relationship works so well.

Denise's crazy relationships are the direct result of how she sees herself. People with a healthy sense of self don't attract, and are not attracted to, addicts and abusers the way some of us do. When addicts and abusers show up in the lives of healthy people, they immediately pick up on the negative vibe and run the other way. They don't invite them over for dinner and casual sex.

Not only is karma not the result of a vindictive Supreme Being, but the events that we label as "bad" have the potential to launch our lives into new directions. There may be lessons to be learned, people to meet, and sacred places to be visited. Sometimes it's those sudden explosions in our lives that give us the momentum to burst forth in brilliance.

Many years ago, my ex-husband Ray and I were both laid off within a day of each other a week before Christmas. We worked for two totally different companies, but within 24 hours we both found ourselves unexpectedly unemployed. Bad karma? Heck, no!

It was that unforeseen "tragedy" that sent the two of us 2200 miles west into the Arizona desert. Then our addictions flared and eventually our marriage collapsed. Bad karma? Nope! The insanity of that relationship spurred me on to get sober and to begin a new life.

A couple of years later, my friend Eileen, asked me out to dinner and the rest is history. We've been in love ever since. Had I not lost that job in Atlanta (and let me tell you, it was a *lousy* job and one I didn't do it very well), I would have never met the woman that amplifies my life's Joy!

I have learned to trust the process, no matter what happens. Karma isn't what causes good and bad things to happen. Karma is what we make of what happens. It's our "experience of the experience" that makes it the tragedy or triumph.

When life throws you a curve, lean into it! Be willing to see things differently and suddenly Karma will slingshot you to unimaginable heights! It's not about what you've done in the past. It's about how you choose to view the present. And tell the Cosmic

Karmic Council of the Misery Conspiracy to take a hike! You won't get coal in your stocking! I promise!

Chapter 22:
Got Butterflies?

One of the things that I've discovered in my journey is that we have the power to transform the weapons of the Misery Conspiracy into tools for Peace. We can take situations, like acts of violence that start out creating pain or upset, turn them around and use them to help people come together in community. We can convert a meth lab into a community center (without the drugs). We can use the heartbreak of September 11 as a reminder to be more respectful and compassionate to other people.

When I was taking public speaking courses in college, I found another example of this transformative process. As I started my first class, I was nervous. I was always a shy kid growing up. The thought of speaking in front of a group of people terrified me. Fortunately, I was blessed with a wonderful professor who really understood the dynamics of public speaking.

Early in the course, the professor told us that it is normal to have butterflies in the stomach when giving a speech. The nervous energy is a natural result of being in a situation where the outcome is important, but uncertain. It is the same nervous energy you might feel if a family member did not arrive home on time, but you had no way of finding out if they were safe. Or if you are waiting to hear about the results of a job interview or a mid-term exam, you get that feeling in the pit of your stomach like you just ate a hyperactive lizard. Yeah, that's nervousness!

"So," you are thinking, "the nervousness is normal, but how do you get rid of it?" The answer is, you don't! If you paid attention in physics class (the only course in college that I flunked, by the way), you may recall that the Law of the Conservation of Energy states that energy cannot be created or destroyed, but it can change form.

Your nervous energy is there. It's dancing around in your stomach (the lizard and the butterflies are having a rave). You cannot force it to go away. Any attempts to do so will just make you more nervous. But there is an alternative.

The solution, according to my professor, is not to get rid of the butterflies, but rather to teach them to fly in formation. In other words, since you are stuck with this energy, put it to work.

When I am giving one of my presentations, I use that energy to give a dramatically more powerful speech. I'll pound the podium! Maybe I'll shout a slogan or reach out and gently touch an audience member on the shoulder! I may even dance a jig (please don't ask me to do it at my book-signing)! I'll try whatever I think will give my speech more flair, all the while making good use of that nervous energy.

When I went to make my first speech, I was terrified. I had been assigned to talk about the tragedies of poverty in the inner city. I had done my research. I had practiced my presentation until I knew it forwards, backwards and in Klingon. But the walk to the lectern felt like I was climbing the gallows steps. My knees shook as I began my introduction.

Then I remembered what my professor told me and re-channeled that energy into my voice. The impact of the speech was so powerful that a few of my class members were moved to tears. And to top it off, I wasn't nervous. I felt exhilarated and powerful. You, too, can do this.

If you're looking for a job and you're nervous about an interview, turn that nervous energy upside down and use it to embolden your presentation. If you're on a first date, use that energy to make your date's experience as wonderful as possible. If a loved one is overdue and it's too early to call the hospitals, use the time to clean house! Find ways to redirect any negative energy into a more positive and useful form.

Got butterflies? Then teach that energy fly!

Chapter 23:
No! No! You Can't Take God Away From Me!

Christianity describes us as "the body of the Christ", the embodiment or expression of the Divine. *A Course in Miracles* calls us the "Thoughts of God" and states that "thoughts do not leave their source". We are intrinsically and eternally connected to the Consciousness of Love at our most fundamental levels. We are the One Self.

While our connection to our Spiritual Source cannot be severed, the Misery Conspiracy will do everything it can to lead you to believe that it can. It will tell you that God hates you. It will tell you that God has turn His back on you. It will distract you with thousands of things that it tells you are more important than Love and Serenity.

A minister once asked me, "If God is ever-present, but you feel alone and isolated, who moved?" It is a very poignant question. When we feel separated from our Divine Source, it is always us who turned away from the Truth. And the good news is that we can always turn back, whenever we realize what we did.

There was a time in my life when I was told differently. The defenders of misery told me that God hated me and considered me an abomination. People who claimed to be in God's "little club" turned their back on me, and at a time when I really needed support. It was one of the darkest times of my life, and yet it also taught me one of the most crucial lessons I needed to learn.

I know that there are some people who are born knowing who they are and into which categories they belong. I wasn't one of them. For reasons I still do not fully understand, I was born with a conflict between my plumbing and my wiring. The doctor saw that there was a problem when I was born and did a little surgical procedure to "correct" the problem. Unfortunately, he "corrected" the wrong way.

I grew up with a male body, but always identified as female. Not something I chose or would wish on anyone! As a matter of survival (I had an aversion to getting the snot beat out of me), I learned to play the part of a boy, but it was always an act. I kept hoping as I grew that if I tried hard enough, if I prayed hard enough, if I acted sincerely enough, and if I saw enough therapists, somehow the conflict would go away. It didn't.

When I was in my mid-20s, the conflict became so great that I turned to alcohol and other compulsive behaviors to avoid the feelings. But I eventually hit bottom and realized that I had no other choice if I wanted to stay alive. I had to make changes so that my outside matched my insides.

It was not an act of immorality or of weak character. It was an act of compassion towards myself. And when I made this choice to honor my True Self, the compulsive drinking and other behaviors went away. But even as the conflict within started to abate, my conflict with the outside world exploded!

I lost my family, my friends, my home, and my job. At the time, I was attending and actively involved with a very conservative church (in the hopes that all that praying and singing and Scripture-reading would "cure" me). When I tried to explain to the minister what I had been through and what I was doing to take care of myself, he showed me the door. He told me that God had no room for me in "His Kingdom". I went away heartbroken. I was later kicked out of two other churches for the same reasons.

I struggled with this for about a month. *Why did the thought of coming into my much-delayed womanhood bring me Peace and a sense of Oneness with the Divine? And yet at the same time, why did those who claimed to speak for God want nothing to do with me?* I prayed for God to speak to me, to show me which road to go down. And the response that I got back was, "To thine own Self be True. I am with you always!"

In that moment, I realized that these ministers (and everyone else who had turned their back on me) were within their rights to choose who they wanted in their "club". But they could never take away my relationship with Source of Unconditional Love. Just because they claimed God hated me didn't make it true. God doesn't care about gender. He cares a great deal about our openness to Love.

And so I began a difficult, yet rewarding, journey of spirit and gender exploration. For a very long time, I had almost nothing, as I struggled to re-build a life from scratch. But one thing I always had was my Higher Power, guiding me gently and lovingly through all of the pain and rejection. And eventually, I found a community of loving, open-minded people; a chosen family of friends who celebrate the woman I've become.

My purpose for sharing this with you is not to stir up controversy or shock you. It is to remind you that no one can take God away from you. No one has the ability to make the Consciousness of Unconditional Love withdraw that Love from you. That would be contrary to Its Nature. You are connected to your Divine Source at your most fundamental levels. You can ignore it. You can deny it. But the one thing you can't do with your relationship with your Source is break it. It's permanent.

You need no intermediary to talk to God. You don't need a priest. You don't need a medium. You don't need a Ouija board, or a crystal, or a prayer mala. Just open your mind to the One Self. Open your Spirit to the universal flow of Love. Breathe it in and let it pass on through to those around you. This is Heaven.

Section Three:
Cracking Open
That Spiritual Toolbox

Chapter 24:
Turning Off Autopilot and
Turning On Conscious Creation

In addition to other purposes, your mind serves as a toolbox. It is where we keep our collection of spiritual tools. When I talk about spiritual tools, you don't have to go looking for your tool belt or your tape measure. You don't need to go looking for your 108-bead prayer mala or your golden crucifix or your multi-version, parallel translation Bible with built-in Concordance.

All of those are fine, but when *I* mention spiritual tools, I'm talking about Power Tools not designed by Black and Decker or published by Zondervan. I'm talking prayer, meditation, service work, manifesting and other spiritual processes to put you in conscious contact with your own Divine nature.

A few years back, I had my own business designing jewelry. Yes, I was a girl with a torch! My designs were rather innovative. Perhaps too innovative! My pieces weren't the lightweight, mass-produced stuff from Hong Kong that you see in department stores. They were big, bold and edgy. And I had dreams of being the next "Big Thing". I imagined celebrities showing off my latest creations on the way to hip New York parties.

Then the economy went belly up after the September 11th attacks and demand for my work dropped off significantly. I hired a business coach and read books on marketing. They suggested, in addition to my marketing efforts, that I continue to visualize what success would look like to me. They told me to cut out pictures of what I thought success looked like and to glue them to my workshop walls. And this I did. But sales continued to slump and the one gallery representing my work closed their doors. I guess things were bad for a lot of people.

Not long after I gave up on my career as a world famous jeweler, the concept of consciously creating one's day became a very popular topic in spiritual/metaphysical circles these days. Dr. Joe Dispenza and Ramtha discussed it in the movie, *What the Bleep Do We Know?* The spiritual text, *A Course in Miracles,* dedicates an entire chapter to it. Dr. Wayne Dyer mentions it in his book *Intention.*

We create our day all the time, but we are usually running on autopilot, which tends to be set to a negative, fear-based level that we learned from the Misery Conspiracy. All of this crap shows up in our life and we think the Universe is out to get us. You know, that whole "bad karma" thing again. In reality, the Universe is simply reflecting our own negatively creative thoughts. So if we don't like what we're seeing, it's time to turn off the autopilot and switch to consciously creating our day and our lives.

Consciously creating our day boils down to taking time each morning to redirect our thought process and to visualize how we want our day to unfold and what we want to attract into our lives. We have the potential to dramatically influence the direction of our lives by focusing on what we want to happen and how we will respond to it. We have the power to physically manifest anything we can conceive, given sufficient focus and intention.

But this begs the question: if creating one's day is such an effective tool, why didn't it work for me in my jewelry business? After all, I followed the directions that I was given. I covered my workshop wall with cutout photos of cars and houses and Oprah Winfrey. I visualized making *tons* of sales and making *tons* of money and becoming goldsmith to the stars. But nothing happened! What went wrong?

In the book *Ask and It Is Given*, Abraham explains that visualizing is only half of the equation. The other half is allowing. In other words, we have to see the Universe as abundant and to see ourselves as worthy recipients of that abundance. We have to be open to the process at our deepest levels. Feelings of unworthiness and guilt block the flow of abundance because we are effectively telling the Universe, "Yeah, I want it, but I don't deserve it. I would really like it, but it will never happen." We don't realize what a self-fulfilling prophecy that becomes.

When I was running my jewelry business, I felt guilty when someone bought my work, as if I hadn't earned the money. Is that crazy or what? I was convinced deep in my mind that my work was somehow inferior because I made it. I caught myself subtly talking people out of buying my work, acting apologetic for charging a reasonable price for the time and effort I put into it. This blocked my manifesting my dreams.

Other forms further blocked the flow of abundance in my life. I was desperate for cash. Desperation always denies abundance. I was also terrified of cold-calling galleries to get them to show my jewelry. As much as I loved working with stone and metal, the selling end of my business was suffering due to my fear. Even my visualization exercises were fearful and filled with desperation. And I wonder why my business fizzled?

As much as I wanted money and success, I had a deep seated belief that I wouldn't get them and that I didn't deserve them. Effectively, I was making requests and then telling the Universe, "Never mind. Don't bother." The result was that I manifested what I expected to get: nothing!

I thought at the time that if I just named what I wanted, then somehow, I would get what I was desperate for. When we come from a place where we see ourselves as somehow "not enough" and the universe as offering limited resources for the lucky few, then what we get is "not enough" and limited. And that is exactly what I got.

When we consciously create our day, we start by changing the nature of our thoughts from fearful to loving. We take time to see the Universe as abundant rather than limited. We see ourselves as deserving of that abundance. It helps to see this abundance coming to us as the result of our own generosity to others. The Universe always responds to our attitude towards ourselves and others. Generosity towards others draws generosity to us. Selfishness towards others will be repaid in kind.

As an emerging writer, I visualized not just selling books or booking speaking engagements, but focused on the sharing of my wisdom and contributing to the Joy and Peace of people that I was reaching out to. I let go of a constricted, limited Universe and opened myself to the abundance of the Universe. I saw myself as a vital part of the flow of unconditional love and generosity. I learned to trust the process. Without the limitations of fear and desperation, I found opportunities falling into my lap. People who needed to hear my message were drawn to me.

Taking time each morning to focus on becoming more loving and less judgmental is tremendously powerful. A generous, giving attitude is just as contagious as a selfish, grabby attitude, but with opposite results. Both have a dramatic effect on how the world shows up for us. As I have changed my own attitude towards the Universe, I have been amazed at how abundance and wealth in all forms shows up, often in unexpected ways.

Creating one's day doesn't mean challenges won't arise. But when "bad" things happen, we are less likely to be thrown by them if we have started our day with an intentional focus on the positive. We are calmer and better able to assess our options and determine the best course of action when we have prepared ourselves mentally and spiritually ahead of time. And more likely than not, these challenges turn into boosts for our individual journeys.

Tomorrow morning, as soon as you can remember, take a few moments to focus on letting go of fears and judgments, and then open your mind to receive all the Love and abundance (in whatever form) that is available to you today. Focus on what actions you will take today and imagine yourself surrounded by golden light while doing them. You will discover a whole new way to create your day.

Chapter 25:
Dumping Willpower for Willingness

In 2006, I celebrated 10 years of sobriety. Sobriety birthdays (as such anniversaries are often called) are funny things, especially the big ones such as the one year, five year, ten year and 20 year birthdays. My feelings about them are mixed. Every year when my sobriety birthday comes around, I am greeted by friends with congratulations and adulations. They say that I must have great willpower and that I'm an inspiration.

While the support of friends is appreciated (essential, really), recovering alcoholics or addicts know that staying sober has nothing to do with willpower. If I had any willpower, I wouldn't have been an alcoholic. I'm just a drunk; a drunk who was and is willing.

It is willingness, not willpower, that allows alcoholics and addicts to stop using. The 12 Steps of Alcoholics Anonymous are filled with references to willingness, both direct and indirect. Step One asks us to be *willing* to admit that we have a problem. The second step states that we are *willing* to believe that a power greater than ourselves can restore us to sanity. Our *willingness* to turn our lives over to the care of God, our *willingness* to make an inventory of our past and present behaviors, and our *willingness* to make amends to those we have harmed are all crucial parts of the recovery process.

As I stated before, it took a suicide attempt before I was willing to see that I had a problem. I had been lost in an abusive relationship for years with no idea how to get out. I kept hoping that if I was just nice enough and loving enough and understanding enough, that somehow my then-husband Ray would respond in kind. In my desperation to be loved, I became very clingy and manipulative, only to be rebuffed by Ray's cruel words and actions. According to him, everything wrong in his world was my fault.

A healthy person would have left him long ago, but I was anything but healthy. All I could see from my limited perspective was a list of reasons why I needed to stay. I constantly reminded myself that, because my name was on our apartment lease, I was locked into paying my half of the rent. I couldn't afford to pay rent there and at a new place as well. I was also afraid of what he might try to do if I did leave. When cornered, Ray could be unpredictable.

To cope with this unbearable situation, I would sneak off to bars and drink myself into oblivion. I was desperate for human warmth, even if it was the illusory companionship of my fellow barflies. Under the influence of loneliness and booze, we commiserated with each other our individual nightmares.

The truth is that I didn't have a drinking problem; I had a stopping problem. I was good at drinking. It was stopping at one or two drinks that I found impossible. Each time, I found myself falling-off-the-barstool drunk. It was a miserable way to live, but I was so lonely and so filled with despair that I was powerless to stop. I could hear the time bomb of my life ticking down. In my mind, I counted down with it, like a crowd counting down the last seconds of a basketball game. I longed for whatever oblivion could bring me.

So one night, after my husband had raged at me and gone off to the bars for his latest one-night stand, I decided that I had had enough. I was tired of living in fear all of the time. I made my way to the medicine cabinet and took two aspirin, chasing them down with a shot of Irish whiskey. And then I took two more aspirin. And two more. And two more after that, until I had taken three dozen aspirin, along with half a bottle of whiskey. I had given up. I had become so traumatized that I no longer cared about living. I just wanted to stop the pain. I curled up into a ball on the living room floor and cried myself to sleep for what I hoped was the last time.

The next morning, when Ray found me on the floor, he rushed me to the emergency room. For the next several hours, I was monitored continuously by the ER staff, while I tried to make sense of my out-of-control life.

What was wrong with me? What was I going to do about my life? I had no answers. I was in a state of mental collapse. This was my moment of surrender, my moment of willingness. I prayed for direction; not to God specifically, but to whatever Higher Mind might hear my cries.

Before the suicide, I had prayed to God, asking Him to help me make my husband love me. If God had said anything in response, I didn't hear it. After the suicide attempt, my prayers were less specific. "To whoever's listening, I give up. I'm willing to try anything. I just want Peace."

It was this willingness more than anything else that saved me. I was *willing* to consider a new perspective. I was *willing* to try anything to have a different life. I was *willing* to recognize that not everything about my situation was Ray's fault. I was *willing* to admit I had a problem.

This was the key that unlocked the door to hope and to healing and to radical transformation. Up to this point, I had relied on my own mental resources, but they had betrayed me time after time. Now, I had given up on willpower and chosen willingness instead.

I still had no answers. But in the circle of Alcoholics Anonymous, Al-Anon and other 12-Step programs, I began to find them. I found a new understanding of God, which was very different from the judgmental, vindictive version I had grown up with. Through the sharing of others' stories, the guidance of my sponsor and the application of the tools of my recovery program, I discovered a wisdom and serenity that is beyond what words can describe. I found it *only* because I was willing.

A few years later, willingness took on a whole new meaning. Opportunities to help others in desperate need began showing up. In some cases, it required only that I share my story at a meeting.

At other times, much deeper acts of compassion were needed. Whatever I had, whatever was needed, I gave in hope and gratitude. As part of my recovery, I had not only opened myself up to the process, but had made myself available to be part of the process of healing those in my sphere of influence.

Why would I be willing to do these things? Perhaps it's because I am alive due to the generosity of strangers who shared their stories at meetings, and acquaintances who let me stay with *them* rent-free for extended periods of time. Who was I to refuse help to someone else in a similar situation? After all, this is how we heal the world.

Even after ten years of sober living, willingness is still a crucial part of my life. Without it, I could easily revert back to drinking and all of the insane thought processes that go along with it. To stay alive, sober and serene, I must continuously be willing to see things differently. I must be willing to love myself and those around me. I must be willing to connect to the God of my understanding on a regular basis. And I must be willing to be available to serve others when needed.

Willingness isn't simply a tool for alcoholics. If you are not experiencing Joy and Peace and Love right now, willingness can help you get there. It opens the doors that we locked in our attempts to shut ourselves off from our true nature and from God. Willingness removes the blinders that we have put on, and allows us to see new perspectives and new possibilities. Happiness is yours for the taking. Are you willing?

Chapter 26:
I Love You, But Get Out Of My House!

I'll be the first to admit that I can be dull as a watermelon sometimes, when it comes to learning certain life lessons. It's taken me decades to figure out some things that most people seem to know instinctively.

For example, one would think that after finally making a decision to leave my abusive husband, that that would be the end of it. Nope! I went back to him a few months later thinking that somehow all of our problems had magically vanished. After all, I had been in recovery for five whole months! Not that he was in recovery, but surely I alone could make our broken little marriage work. Yeah, right!

In less than a year, I had attempted suicide again (this time with a Vicodin overdose instead of aspirin) and moved out again. Unfortunately, I was back again after a few more months, in one of the lost episodes of "Lifestyles of the Drunk and Disorderly". When I left him for the third and final time, I got an Order of Protection to not only keep him away from me, but to keep me from going back to him...AGAIN. It worked.

One afternoon, after Ray and I had separated for the second time, he called and asked to come over to my apartment to talk things over. He seemed somewhat reasonable over the phone. Still holding onto the dream of a happily-ever-after with him, I agreed to let him in. What can I say? Any lesson not learned the first time will be repeated until it is learned. It was time for my make-up exam!

Less than ten minutes into our conversation, he was back to his usual blaming and shaming behaviors. Suddenly he was waxing malicious about how everything wrong in our relationship was my fault. In the days before my emotional breakdown (or more accurately my *emotional breakthrough*), I would have played the Misery Conspiracy's game of defending myself against ridiculous accusations. But armed with the wisdom of my recovery program, I knew that it's a game that can't be won. So I didn't play. Instead I took responsibility.

Because he was on my turf (or at least in my apartment), I led him to the door and forced him to leave. That was a ground-breaking moment for me. I honored a boundary for the first time in my life. I half expected the skies to open up and for a chorus of cherubim to break in to song. I had to settle for Ray's not-so-melodic pounding on my door.

Setting this boundary didn't make Ray Happy. In fact, he pounded on my door for the next half hour, begging me to let him back in (I half expected him to huff and puff and blow the door down). I thought I'd feel empowered when I set a boundary. Instead, I was scared. No one had warned me about this side effect of setting boundaries.

I called my friend Terri, who was also in recovery. While Ray pounded away at my door, Terri reassured me that I was doing the right thing. This helped get me through the immediate trauma, and paved the way for future boundary setting. Ray eventually got the hint that this little piggy wasn't letting him back in and left.

Sometimes people confuse extending unconditional love to everyone with being doormats to any jerk that comes along. That simply is not the case. We do not need to let anyone abuse us or take advantage of our generosity and compassion in ways that compromise our Joy and Serenity. While everyone is worth loving and is need of love, there are a lot of crazy, dangerous people out there (I used to be one of them). Just because I love you, doesn't mean that I necessarily want you in my kitchen (and vice versa).

When someone behaves inappropriately, the most loving response is often to say, "No, not here!" Not only does it honor your own need for Peace and safety, it sends them a message that may have some issues that need addressing. Ignoring their behavior or allowing them to harm you and others only serves to reinforce their belief that what they are doing is okay. In recovery, we call it "enabling".

Back when I was designing jewelry, I had a friend who was a very talented silversmith. His work had been featured in museums and national magazines. When he was sober, he was a delight to be around. But when he was drunk, which was most of the time, he had all of the appeal of an infected toenail.

So the first time I saw him drunk, I made it clear to him that I do not spend time people that are intoxicated, not even close friends. Of course, drunks are not known for their ability to remembering such things, particularly when they're on a bender. So eventually things between us got...well, UGLY!

Once I picked him up to go to a tradeshow. From his rather fluid and irregular movements, I could tell that he had been drinking (either that or the aliens were activating the chip in his brain). At first, I chose to ignore it. But as I started driving down the road, he reveals a plastic cup filled with what appeared to be soda. My instinct went on high alert and told me that it wasn't just soda in that cup. My instinct was right.

"Jason, are you drinking alcohol in my truck?" I asked him.

"Naw, it's just soda," he slurred. But I could tell from his mannerisms that he was lying. He had a half-lit, skulky look on his face and he wouldn't look me in the eye. So I pulled into a gas station a few miles from his house.

"Jason, look at me!" I demanded. "What are you drinking?" He admitted that there was vodka in the cup and that he'd been drinking most of the morning. What a surprise!

"Jason, you are my friend and I care very much for you. But I do not allow alcohol in my truck, and you know this. You're going to have to get out."

He just sat there. I repeated my demand a few times, but he didn't move. So I had to go through the humiliation (his humiliation, not mine) of physically dragging a grown, drunk man out of my truck. Let me just say for the record that I'm glad that drunks are really bad at fighting. He took a swing at me, missed (big surprise!), but managed to connect solidly with the side of my truck. In the end, I drove on to the tradeshow without him. He got to walk home with his cup of soda and booze.

Kicking him out of the truck and leaving him to walk home drunk might sound harsh. But the fact is that he invaded my personal space with his alcohol, with full knowledge that I don't allow booze in my truck. He put me at risk for getting charged with violating the open container law. He had no regard for me or the boundaries that I use to keep myself sober. Dumping him at the gas station was my way of honoring my need to be safe. It also served as a reminder to him that his behavior was unacceptable and that maybe he should get some help.

It is said in the 12-Step program that we can either honor our boundaries or we can take care of their feelings. We cannot do both. Ray didn't like it when I set a boundary with him. Jason wasn't too thrilled either. People don't like it when you call them on their crap. Folks are funny that way. Regardless of their reaction, though, the most loving thing that we can do is to set and honor our boundaries. It's like saying, "Get the Hell out of here!" but in a loving way.

How we honor our boundaries can make a big difference in the outcome. I learned this the third and final time I ended up leaving Ray (what can I say; I'm just glad I didn't go back for Round# 4). Like our previous two breakups, there was plenty of drama.

He had moved in with me to the same apartment that I had kicked him out of months before. Despite the fact that he, too, was now in recovery, it didn't take long for things to go squirrelly again. The old routine of avoidance, rage, infidelity and reconciliation picked up almost immediately. I suppose it was like riding a bicycle; a very dysfunctional bicycle.

Eventually the police were called during one of our full-contact screaming matches. I figured that since only my name was on the lease, he would be the one forced to leave. I figured wrong!

Ray told the police that since I had friends that I could stay with (which was true), but that he had no friends (also true, but not my problem), that I should be the one to leave. And to my amazement, the police officers agreed. I was escorted out of my own apartment, put in the back of the police cruiser, and driven to my sponsor's house. Meanwhile, he got to stay in my apartment...but only for one night.

Justice was served the next morning in the form of an Order of Protection, forcing him to move out of the apartment that day. And when he tried to quash the Order, I showed up at the hearing with a long detailed history of his out-of-control, rage-aholic behaviors. I was determined to honor my boundaries and I prevailed.

When we set boundaries the focus should always be on the behavior and not on the person doing the behavior. If during the hearing I had told the judge that I needed the Order of Protection because Ray was a jerk, it might have been quashed. But because I made it about his inappropriate, violent behavior, the judge saw that the Order was needed.

Another thing to keep in mind is that we don't always have the right to demand the offending person leave if we are in common or neutral space, such as a shared apartment or a restaurant. If I had been in Jason's car and he was drinking, I couldn't exactly kick him out of his own car (or drag him out as the case may be). But I could choose to get out of the car myself and honor my boundary that way. That may seem obvious, but sometimes there is the temptation to go from setting boundaries to taking control.

In my final confrontation with Ray, when the police were insisting that I be the one to leave, however unfairly, my best choice was not to take control, but to remove myself from the situation. We only have a right to ask someone to leave if they are in *our* personal space, and if that doesn't work we have to look at alternatives. If we are in their space or in neutral territory, such as a restaurant, or have no way of enforcing the boundaries in our personal space, it's always best to remove *ourselves* from the situation without making a dramatic scene.

I can't demand that my employer not have alcohol at the holiday party. I can make a request, but I have to leave the ultimate decision to whoever is planning the party. Generally, I don't go to parties where alcohol is served. After all, it is my responsibility to avoid situations that put my sobriety at risk.

Setting and honoring boundaries is a great way to put the kibosh on the insanity of the Misery Conspiracy. We see the games being played, and when someone hits the ball to our side of the court, we can let it bounce or roll on by.

When people are inappropriate and out-of-control, we can walk away. We can tell them to take a hike. We can take a stand and say, "I love you, but get out of my house!"

Chapter 27:
Catch and Release

Learning to handle strong emotions is another vital skill in combating the Misery Conspiracy. While emotions are an important part of our life experience, we can run into trouble if they start to run our lives. When left unchecked, emotions can lead us to express our feelings in ways that are harmful to ourselves and others. Similarly, if we just shut down all of our emotions, we shut ourselves off from our Joy, even as misery manages to squeeze its way into our psyche.

One morning I got into my little pick'em up truck on my way to a writer's conference. The day before, my partner Eileen had borrowed my truck to haul something. At the time, I had reminded her to stop for gas, because less than a quarter tank remained in the truck. When I got into my truck the next day, I noticed the fuel gauge. It was not on "E". It was about two inches BELOW "E". That's when the Misery Conspiracy came charging up to "handle" the situation.

I managed to drive around the corner to the nearest gas station and, while I was fueling up, picked up my cell phone. Guess who I called? Yup! Eileen! Any guesses on the tone of my voice? Was I calm and respectful? Are you kidding? No, I was in downtown Blame City! All the while, I was staring blankly at my license plate, which reads (are you ready for this?) AGAPE2U, which in LicenseSpeak means "unconditional love to you".

The point of this story (aside from reminding you to always check your fuel gauge) is that we all get upset from time to time. There is a tendency among some of us to deny this annoying little truth. We would much rather keep those feelings stuffed deep into our subconscious and heavily sedated (because that worked so well for us in the past...not!). But denying and burying our negative feelings is not the answer. They will manifest themselves one way or another if left to their own devices (sneaky little devils aren't they?). That's why I've adopted a "catch and release" program.

Having spent the last decade on an intensive spiritual journey, I have a tendency to avoid any negative emotions because of my hyper-awareness of their destructive nature. I am not alone in this (which is good because I hate to be alone!). A lot of self-help gurus tell us that we should not be angry. We should not be judgmental. We should not be resentful. We should not engage in self-pity, etc. Oh, and we shouldn't "should" on people. Oh darn, I'm doing it again!

To an extent, there is a lot of wisdom in avoiding negative emotions. Many of us who are looking for a better life have made great efforts to root out the negative thought patterns that previously made us so miserable. As a result, we are no longer caught up in the nightmarish drama that once ruled our lives. Yea for us!

However, even the most enlightened of us still get triggered (except me, I NEVER get triggered...yeah, right!) So what do we do with emotions like anger and sadness and resentment when they arise?

Well, I've taken to a "catch and release" program. As many of you may know, "catch and release" is a fishing technique that allows fishermen (and fisherwomen, to be politically correct) to catch fish, but requires the fish to be released back into the water in order to maintain the population. This allows the fisherpersons (okay, now that just sounds silly) to enjoy the sport of fishing without wrecking the local ecosystem.

How does this apply to negative emotions? When a negative emotion arises, we give ourselves permission to feel ("catch") it for a brief period, but then we let go ("release") of it. This approach prevents the hyper-vigilant tendency we may have to suppress any emotion we don't like, while at the same time not leading us back into the Hell of a life ruled by anger, self-pity and fear. This does not mean that we can act out with these emotions in ways that harm ourselves or others. It simply means that we allow ourselves to be in the moment and feel the emotions, and then let go of them, if necessary with help from our Higher Power (i.e. God, our Source, etc.).

So letting yourself feel ticked off for a few moments when someone cuts you off in traffic is cool, but running them off the road...not so cool! In the case of the gas in my truck, allowing myself to feel the frustration was helpful, but calling up my partner and shaming her not filling up the tank was not helpful to either one of us (I apologized to her about 10 minutes later, by the way).

How long you hold onto an emotion before releasing it is an individual decision, and can vary depending on the situation. If you get stuck behind a stalled car during rush hour (can you tell I have issues with driving?), it might be appropriate to feel a bit miffed for a minute or two. Any longer than that and you risk hosting a pity party for one.

The ending of a relationship or the death of a loved one brings up more intense emotions of grief and may require more time and effort to work through. Don't force it, just don't let it re-landscape your world into an emotional swamp complete with mosquitoes the size of a Buick.

Do what you can to prevent negative emotions from arising by re-training your mind with prayer, meditation, journaling, reading inspirational or self-help books, and limiting exposure to negative messages from T.V., movies, music and your mother, who keeps asking you when you're going to make her a grandmother. But when negative emotions arise (and they will!), don't deny them. Don't bury them. Just remember "catch and release"!

Chapter 28:
It's Not Just For Catholics Anymore!

Some spiritual tools, such as creating one's day, are just now coming into the public consciousness. Others, such as prayer and meditation, have been around forever. Some of these classic tools have been discarded as worthless and no longer useful. And yet, perhaps there is a use for them that we just haven't seen.

As a recovering Catholic, I remember going to confession when I was a child. The first time it took me a while just to think of something I needed to confess. Even after fifteen minutes, all I could come up with was that I'd let the air out of Timmy Bradshaw's bicycle tire after he beat me up. What can I say? I was a good kid for a while. Of course, I made up for it later.

For years, the whole confession deal seemed to me so patriarchal and political, as if the Church was simply trying to justify its existence. Why go through a priest, I wondered. Why not talk directly to God? And what purpose does it serve (other than to numb our minds) to say the same old prayers over and over *ad nauseum*? I just didn't get it.

It's funny how our perspective changes over the years. With maturity comes a better understanding of old ways and traditions and the purposes they serve. Such has been the way my view of the confessional has changed.

As I explained in a previous chapter, we are always free to open our hearts directly to God, without the need of a third party. But sometimes it's helpful to talk with someone we can see and touch, whether it's a priest, a therapist or a friend. I've tried talking to my cats, but all I get back is "Clean my litter box!" On second thought, maybe there's a hidden message in that!

The Fourth Step of Alcoholics Anonymous tells alcoholics like me to take an unflinching look at our personal histories. Typically, these histories are written down and may include a retelling of events in our lives that led to our addictive behaviors and how the disease of addiction has caused our lives to go out of control. Once this history or inventory is completed, it is then shared with another person (Step Five), usually one's sponsor who acts as a mentor in recovery.

Like a lot of addicts, I found this process difficult and humbling. While I trusted my sponsor, sharing the ugly details of my history left me feeling naked and exposed. I no longer had the shields of anonymity or denial to hide behind. The brutal truth was out.

The feelings of vulnerability passed, however, and were replaced with the freedom of no longer being burdened under all of the lies, secrecy, and delusions. It's amazing how much energy it takes to hide who we are. I was able to let go of the guilt and shame of my past. And I could take comfort in knowing that my sponsor, too, had had similar struggles. I was not alone.

The use of repeated prayers as a follow up to confessing has also been a part of my recovery process. When we repeat a prayer over and over, we start to see new meanings in it, and learn to apply these insights to the particulars of our lives.

During the early years of my recovery from addiction, my sponsor kept telling me to repeat the Serenity Prayer at least three times a day. Had it been anyone else making the suggestion, I would have told them to stick it where the sun doesn't shine (like Alaska on a warm December night). But I learned from Day One to do what my sponsor told me, no matter how boring or stupid it sounded.

For those not familiar with it, the Serenity Prayer goes like this:

God,

Grant me Serenity to accept the things I cannot change,

Courage to change the things I can,

And Wisdom to know the difference.

Amen.

After saying the Serenity prayer for the hundredth time, I started to see how the words applied to situations in my life. As a compulsive manipulator, I started to see that I cannot change other people's actions or attitudes towards me. I couldn't change how my ex-husband treated me. I couldn't change how my parents saw me. For these things, I needed to ask my Higher Power for Serenity.

I also started to see that it was *up to me* whether I continued to live in an abusive marriage or to find a way to live elsewhere. I started to understand that how I saw people and how I treated them, including the words I used, made a difference in how I was treated. When I responded to the world with fear and anger, I got the same back. When I responded to the world with compassion and acceptance, I got that back too in most cases. So I asked my Higher Power for the courage to change the things I could: my actions and my attitudes.

Finally, I learned to ask for Divine Guidance to understand what, in any given situation, I could change (and how to change it) and what I had no control over. Over time, this Wisdom became more powerful than the old messages of the Misery Conspiracy that had held me hostage for so long. It was a promise of the 12-Step program that eventually, I would instinctively be able to handle situations that used to baffle me. Through the use of this prayer, I have done just that.

Whether you're Catholic or not, find someone with whom you can bare your soul on a regular basis. And then find a prayer such as the Serenity Prayer (or any other prayer that speaks to you), and repeat it at least once times a day. With each repetition, consider how the words apply to your situation. You will be amazed at how the acts of confession and reciting prayers can change your perspective.

Also, take some time to reconsider some traditions from your past that might yet be useful if viewed in a new light. As with the concept of "original sin," sometimes it just takes a new perspective on an old tradition to discover a new spiritual tool.

Chapter 29:
Angry Lesbian Music

At a lot of the jobs I've had, the end of the month is crunch time! All the big bosses want their numbers to be good (to make *their* bosses happy), so they encourage, cajole and threaten the worker bees like me to close every possible deal. Getting through the load of work that suddenly drops on my desk requires that I have just the right music.

Turn on my MP3 player. Slip the ear buds in my ears. Select PLAY MUSIC. Select PLAYLISTS. Scroll down the list. Click on "Angry Lesbian Music". Engage! The sounds of Melissa Etheridge, Ani Di Franco, Sinéad O'Connor, the Indigo Girls, and 10,000 Maniacs surge through my brain like a double shot espresso. Yes, I know that they're not all lesbians, but that's just what I call my playlist. Get over it.

There was a time when "angry lesbian music" was my music of choice 24/7, back when I was a single thirty-something, driving around in my little pick'em up truck (standard dyke issue), smoking Marlboro reds, drinking double-strength coffee and sportin' a leather jacket and a butch pixie haircut. And a lot of the time, I was angry.

Things have changed since then. I'm no longer single. A Buick Park Avenue has replaced my pick'em up truck. I've given up smoking and can no longer fit into my leather jacket (still sportin' the butch pixie haircut). Most importantly, I have realized that while I still love my "angry lesbian music", listening to it all of the time comes with a price. I tend to *stay* angry. I become judgmental and confrontational. I tend to block my own Serenity.

This has less to do with the music itself and more to do with what the music means to me. "Angry lesbian music" represents my rejection of the authoritarian, white-male-Christian-oriented thinking that sees me as unworthy of love. But also includes my resentments towards those who may or may not embody that belief system. And that's where I run into trouble.

I have found the same problems creeping in when I spend too much time listening to the news or worse news-oriented talk shows like "Meet the Press" or "Face the Nation". I hear the partisan, one-sided rhetoric from Democrats and Republicans alike and I want to scream at them all, "You're full of shit! Tell the truth for once! Stop playing games! Stop playing politics. Start acknowledging your part in all of this!"

When I started to see these patterns emerging in myself, I realized that what I was feeding my mind was having an impact on how I saw the world. If I listen to music and news that is dishonest and judgmental, I lose touch with the One Self. The Misery Conspiracy creeps into my thinking. I divide the world in the Us's and the Thems. This is where mindfulness helps.

Mindfulness, or awareness as it's sometimes called, is a tool that is very big in Buddhist traditions. It is the practice of focusing one's consciousness on what you're doing and feeling in this present moment. Becoming consciously aware of what we're doing can point us to issues that have been sitting right under our noses for years. We've just been too busy to notice them.

I can watch the news with its endless opera of murders, war stories, political corruptions and celebrity trials. Or I can watch a documentary about the wonders of marine life. Each has a different effect on my mood and thought process.

I can read about the latest fashion fads in Cosmo (with its airbrushed photos of anorexic models) or I can read about how to change my perspective in Marianne Williamson's latest book. I can listen to the hottest hip-hop hits (with its pimp glam culture), or I can listen to more meditative music. Again, what I let into my brain can either increase my connection to Love or block it.

The choices are endless, and it isn't about one being bad and another being good. It's about becoming aware that some choices empower the Misery Conspiracy, while others free us from it and strengthen our Spirit, instead. "It's just choices and consequences," as we say in the 12-Step programs.

In my own journey, I came to this realization and decided it was time to reprogram my mind. There are times in our lives when listening to "angry lesbian music" or "anti-authoritarian rap" helps to get us through difficult periods. It reminds us that we are not alone in our suffering. That was why I listened to it for a very long time.

But eventually, I needed something more spiritually nourishing. Now I listening more often than not to audio CD's from Eckhart Tolle, Dr. Wayne Dyer, the Dalai Lama and many others. This helps me refocus my attention onto how we are all connected, rather than how we seem to be divided.

I am not suggesting that Eckhart Tolle is a better person than Melissa Etheridge, or that Melissa's music is of little value. I love them both and am grateful for how each of them has enriched my life. But I can either wallow in stories of betrayal, or I can learn how to reclaim my Joy. I have chosen to reprogram my mind for the better.

What messages are you allowing into your life, even if it's for entertainment purposes? The old programmer's slogan of "Garbage in, garbage out" holds true for entertainment as well. If much of what you watch, listen to, and read contains the messages of the Misery Conspiracy, you can be sure it's having a negative effect on your life.

For a week, make a list of the movies and TV shows you watch, the computer games you play, the music and radio programs you listen to, and include the kind of messages they offer. Write down why you are engaging in these forms of entertainment. What need is it fulfilling in you? How do you feel afterwards? And is it how you really want to feel? If not, it's time for a change in your entertainment diet. It's time to become more mindful of what you're putting in your mind.

Chapter 30:
Gratitude for Q-Tips

A few years ago, I gave my first speech at Toastmasters. It went very well and I received some very helpful feedback. After the meeting, one of my fellow members told me that it wasn't necessary to thank the audience at the end of my speech. While the suggestion was well intentioned, I respectfully disagreed. It may not be a required part of the Toastmaster etiquette, but it's necessary to me for my own reasons.

One of the reasons I have stayed sober for so long is gratitude. When I was still drinking, I was filled with resentments. I resented my parents for turning their backs on me when I came out of the closet. I resented my ex-husband for his abusive behavior. I resented the world for a myriad of offenses. I was just full of judgments towards everyone, including myself. And I was miserable. What a surprise!

But in recovery, I learned that my resentments and judgments contributed to my drinking and to my misery. To stay sober and to find Serenity, I needed to dump my resentments and start focusing on gratitudes. I didn't think I had much to be grateful for at the time. I was separated from my husband, renting a lousy room from a bizarro family (we're talking motorcycles in the living room and lice everywhere!), and struggling to pay my bills.

But I was sober and I could be grateful for that. And at least I had someplace to sleep at night. I had a decent job. I was in good health. I could be grateful for all of that. And by becoming grateful, I was able to get out of my self-pity. Gratitude led me to help others get sober. It led me to reach out to people in need.

My life now centers on gratitude because it keeps me sober and helps me fend off self-destructive attitudes. It's a matter of survival. With nearly every post on my blog, I include a list of things that I am grateful for. It can be anything from another day of sobriety to my spouse Eileen to the invention of Q-Tips (because their just so darn useful). What I'm grateful for can be as profound or as mundane as I like, so long as I am grateful.

Focusing on what is good in my life keeps me in a positive mindset and acts as a spiritual fuel that keeps me going through each day. So it may not be necessary to an audience member that I thank them for listening to me, but it is very necessary to me to express my gratitude. Otherwise, it would be so easy to slip back into self-pity and resentments.

Even in difficult times, I have found a lot to be grateful for. After the 9/11 attacks, things got financially tough for Eileen and me. We lost our business and we almost lost our home. When Thanksgiving rolled around, I was grateful that we still had a home and the means to pay for it, even though I was desperately searching for a permanent job. I can still remember what it was like to live with my ex-husband and not to have a safe place to sleep at night.

Gratitude changes the direction of our thinking. It needs to be a part of our daily routine, because the Misery Conspiracy is always working to subvert our Joy. To counteract this, making a "gratitude list" realigns our thinking to Love rather than fear. Whether you post your daily gratitude list on your blog or write it in a gratitude journal or just scribble it on the back of a grocery list, it's essential to do it.

Even when dealing with catastrophic situations, there is always something to be grateful for. It may take some introspection, but if we are willing, we can find at least something to lift our spirits. Maybe you can't pay your bills, but for the moment you still have some food in the cabinet, even if it's just stale bread and peanut butter. Some people don't even have that. Or maybe you're in the final stages of a devastating cancer, but you have at least one person who will sit with us through our chemo treatment, even if it's just the crabby nurse with the bad breath and icy hands.

The next time you're in a sour mood, feeling sorry for yourself, or starting to suspect that the Universe is out to destroy you, take ten minutes to make a list of things you're grateful for.

Better yet, make it a habit to start every day with making a list of three to five things you are grateful for, and don't repeat items from one day to the next. Stretch your imagination to think of things you've taken for granted. That will send the Misery Conspiracy running for cover!

Chapter 31:
Go Soak Your Head!

We hear a lot about how important it is to meditate. But how many of us actually take the time to do it on a regular basis? Not as many as need it, I can tell you that!

Why is that? Yes, it takes practice to quiet the mind. But if we understood how wonderfully healing it can be, we wouldn't hesitate to put in the sitting time.

In 1924, President Franklin Roosevelt went down to Warm Springs, Georgia, to soak in the warm spring water to counteract the paralyzing effects of polio. Long before the presidential motorcade pulled up, it was believed that soaking in these springs can have a significant healing effect on the body. A few years after his first visit, President Roosevelt founded the Roosevelt Warm Springs Institute for Rehabilitation, which is still in operation today.

Meditation is like a spiritual soak in healing waters. It is very powerful in counteracting the painful and paralyzing effects of a world run by the Misery Conspiracy. Like the hydrotherapy used by President Roosevelt, the healing process of meditation is a very passive one. You can't force the healing to take place. You simply must allow it to happen at a natural pace. There is a surrendering that must occur in order to achieve maximum results.

I hear people complain that they can't meditate; that their minds are just too busy, or worse, that their schedules are too busy. When that's the case, their need to meditate is even greater.

In fact, the Journal of Clinical Psychiatry has reported that studies show Transcendental Meditation (one of many forms of meditation) can actually help people with Attention Deficit and Hyperactivity Disorder, as well as Asberger's Syndrome and mood disorders. It treats not only the symptoms, but the causes as well, without the side-effects caused by stimulants and other drugs.

If people with ADHD can meditate, surely you can! Just take the time to practice regularly and allow the learning process to improve your skill level. No one is born knowing how to ski or how to play the piano (aside from a few savants). These are things that we have to engage in regularly in order to gain proficiency. We have to allow for mistakes. We have to let go of our attachment to perfection.

Another point I'd like to make about meditation is that, even if you are a Buddhist monk or nun, you can't engage in it all the time. If President Roosevelt had spent all of his time soaking in Warm Springs, he would have looked like one of the singing California Raisins. We might have nicknamed him President Raisin-velt.

He had to balance his soak time with the time he spent performing his presidential duties. As spiritual practitioners and residents of this physical Universe, we have to balance our time between doing our daily spiritual soak and engaging with the world.

The Buddha Shakyamuni spent years meditating to gain enlightenment, but not for enlightenment's sake. His goal was always to find a way to end the suffering of others. When he finally reached enlightenment, he took what he had learned and put it into practice. He taught it to others. He reached out to those in need of his wisdom and shared it. Had he not, his lessons would have died when his body died. And who would that have served?

Spiritual practice is often a practice of balance, of finding the Middle Way, as the Buddha called it. We must discipline and heal our minds by soaking them in the healing waters of meditation. And then we must share that healing with those around us.

We do this by improving how we interact with family members and co-workers. We do this by practicing Compassion with those in need and Forgiveness with those who have wronged us. Not only does this practice help others, but it firms up these lessons in our own minds. As *A Course in Miracles* states frequently, we learn what we teach.

Set aside time every day to give your mind a spiritual soak, even if it's just five minutes in the restroom at work. Then put the benefits of the meditation to work in the world around you. This is how we counteract the effects of the Misery Conspiracy and gain our own enlightenment.

Chapter 32:
The Gift of Asshole Angels

Some of the tools in our spiritual toolbox are not things to do. They are people. They can be friends, therapists and mentors. They can be 12-Step sponsors, ministers, or a stranger on the bus. They can also be asshole angels!

We all have people in our lives who manage to push our hot buttons. Maybe it's our mother, or our partner or our boss, or the distracted drivers on the highway. My mentor, Kaay, refers to these people as "asshole angels." They are one of those gifts that Life sends us that test our patience and the limits of our compassion. We wonder whose idea it was to bring them into our life. It's not until much later that we discover why.

Yes, it's easy to see how they can be assholes. They make us angry. They waste our time. They make our lives miserable. Have a few people in your life that fit that description? Thought so! But you're wondering how these assholes could also be angels. Yes, I wondered that too when Kaay told me about this concept.

My dear friend Lupe used to own a small Mexican bakery with her ex-husband Eduardo. Even though they were divorced, they were able to remain friends. But relations between them became strained when Deborah, the owner of the craft store next door, started coming over every day to flirt with Eduardo on her lunch break.

What bothered Lupe wasn't the fact that Eduardo was interested in another woman. He had dated several women since their divorce. It never upset Lupe. But when Deborah came over, she totally ignored Lupe. She wouldn't even acknowledge her when she walked in. Instead, Deborah flirted and giggled in her revealing sun dresses, as she sat entranced by Eduardo's Latin machismo.

Additionally, and as much as she hated to admit it, the fact that Deborah was Anglo added to her upset. While she no longer cared about Eduardo as a romantic partner, Deborah was an outsider to the traditional Mexican values that Lupe and Eduardo shared. Lupe felt Eduardo was betraying their culture by flirting with the gringa.

As this situation dragged on for a month or so, Lupe's resentments towards Deborah grew. Then one morning as Deborah bounced in with her bleached blonde hair and her Botox smile, Lupe managed to catch Deborah's eye. For just an instant, Lupe saw through Deborah's mask of feigned youthfulness. She saw a frightened little girl, desperate to be loved. Suddenly, Lupe abandoned her judgments of Deborah. She felt ashamed of resenting her, as memories of how Lupe herself struggled for her father's (and later her husband's) affection flooded her soul. Deborah was Lupe's asshole angel.

Despite their special skill to drive us nuts, these asshole angels are often our best teachers. They show us the limits that we've set on our willingness to Love. We think, "I'd love them if they did this or if they had a better attitude." Okay, maybe not. More likely we're thinking, "This person is such a jerk. I hate him/her." We don't realize that by setting limits on our Love, we are setting limits on our Joy.

The lesson from these rather unwitting teachers is this: if we look past their actions and attitudes, if we become willing to Love them, then we can experience a profound Peace. It may seem unfamiliar and strange at first, because the Misery Conspiracy doesn't want us to experience Peace.

The Misery Conspiracy says, "This person doesn't deserve to be loved. They deserve to be punished! Someone should do something about them." That is fear-based thinking and will never bring Joy.

Instead, let us listen to the Voice of Love-based thinking, what some people call God or the Holy Spirit or Buddha! If we listen, we will learn that withholding Love for any reason results in fear. Extending Love, regardless of circumstances, will always result in Peace and Joy.

Even after Lupe let go of her resentments, Deborah still ignored her and continued to flirt with Eduardo like a school girl. Lupe just closed her eyes and silently blessed her asshole angel, and a few months later, Deborah started to acknowledge Lupe and in time engaged her in conversation.

Let us be grateful to the asshole angels in our lives. They are our teachers and our healers. They show us how to Love. What a wondrous gift! And by being grateful, we can heal them, as well.

One last word about asshole angels; just as others are asshole-angels to us, odds are that we are someone else's asshole angel, too. How wonderful, eh? That's what I call a cleverly crafted spiritual tool!

Chapter 33:
The Power of a Smile

It's 5:36 p.m., and I run into the local supermarket on my way home from work. I really don't want to be here. The store is crowded. I'm tired and hungry. Unfortunately, there's nothing to eat at home. So here I am, pushing the cart that pulls to the right (how is it that I always get the broken one?), trying not to crash into my fellow grumpy shoppers. It is times like this that my ego tends to get into full gear. *Can't that mother control her kids? Why can't this store get any decent produce? Did you see what that woman was wearing? Why are there only three registers open when the lines stretch all the way to the meat counter?*

I really don't enjoy being this way. Being negative and judgmental doesn't make me Happy. Complaining about things doesn't make me Happy. In fact, all of this whining is just making me feel worse. After all, it's not like I plan to be here all night. I just have to put a few things in my cart, pay for them, and continue home. It will only take 30 minutes at the most and then I can relax. Why do I feel the need to take an essentially neutral experience and turn it into a nightmare?

It is then that I am reminded of the real reason I here. It doesn't have anything to do with groceries. Every situation in my life is an opportunity to let go of my judgments and fear. Every encounter is filled with possibility to heal myself, and ultimately the world. I just have to be willing to see my circumstances differently. I have to be willing to choose love instead of fear.

When I am willing, it is like a switch being triggered in my spirit. Suddenly, I am no longer the miserable grump that walked into the store.

One of the practices I have developed to help me overcome my negativity is smiling at people. It's a great defense against the negativity of the Misery Conspiracy. Especially when I am in places where I would rather not be, such as the grocery store, waiting in line at the Department of Motor Vehicles, and on the bus, smiling is like a silver bullet.

When I smile, my goal is to help the person I'm smiling at to realize that there is someone on this planet that truly cares about who they are and what they are feeling. I give them a smile that they can see in my eyes and feel in their heart. And here is the kicker: I smile at EVERYBODY. That includes the people that the Misery Conspiracy tells me don't deserve a smile; mothers with screaming kids, gangbangers wearing their colors with their hats cocked, and homeless people begging for change. When I no longer listen to the Misery Conspiracy to decide who deserves love and who doesn't, I am better able to connect with everyone at a deeper level.

Not everyone smiles back, of course, but a lot of people do. Even the ones that don't smile still feel the effects of my love, if only at a subconscious level. Love is just that infective. These non-smilers (hey! I just made up a word!) are also the ones that need it most. People who don't smile back are burdened by a low self-esteem. They see themselves as unloved and unlovable. Smiling at them with such heartfelt enthusiasm tells them that they are loved, that they are deserving of love. If enough people do the same, they start to believe it's true.

Smiling at the mother with the screaming kids reminds her that she is not alone. It lets her know that she can find Peace amidst the semi-controlled chaos of her life. Perhaps my smile will help her be just a little more understanding of her kids' boundless energy. Perhaps she will find a way to channel their energy in a slightly more positive way as the result of my honoring her.

By smiling at the homeless man, I recognize his humanity and our common need to be loved. I may give him some spare change, a 20-dollar bill or just a smile. The money alone can change little. But the warmth of a smile may give him the courage to transform his life for the better. If he has a drinking problem, perhaps an understanding smile can let him know that I, too, have fought a bitter struggle against alcohol and emerged victorious.

Smiling at the gangbanger has the power to dissolve the fear and isolation that led him to seek companionship in the deadly world of street gangs. It shows that I do not fear him, but that I do love him. A smile could give him pause enough to reconsider some of his life choices. If others smile at him too, with the same courage and compassion, he could find a more loving way to live.

To some, the possibilities created by a simple smile may seem overly optimistic. It is such a little thing, smiling. Yet it is often a small change that can lead to bigger changes. It can be the straw that breaks the ego's back; the tiny crack in the dam that leads to the flood of emotion, allowing for a transformative healing. A spiritual awakening doesn't always start with a bang. Often it is a slow realization that the things that we have been doing no longer serve us the way they used to. It is the accumulation of little reminders that gradually bring us to this point of re-birth. A sincere smile from a stranger can become one of those transformative reminders.

The next time you find yourself fighting your way through the supermarket or twiddling your thumbs in your doctor's waiting room, try smiling at the people around you. Don't be afraid to make eye contact. These are human beings like you, not pit bulls. They are tired and hungry and uncomfortable just like you. And like you, there are a lot of other places they would rather be at the moment. So why not give them a smile? Not a smirk. Not a grimace. Give them a genuine smile that they can see in your eyes and feel in your heart. They will feel better. You will feel better. All of a sudden, the nightmare is a little less, well...nightmarish. Smile!

Chapter 34:
The Triple Whammy of Love

Throughout history, the number three has been considered a number of power and of balance. The Pagans had their Triple Goddess (commonly referred to as the Maiden, Mother and Crone). The Christians have the Holy Trinity (Father, Son and Holy Spirit). And let's not forget the Dumas' Three Musketeers (Porthos, Athos and that other guy) or television's classic threesome, the Three Stooges (Moe, Larry, Shemp, Curly and Joe...okay, there were five of them, so what?). Last but not least, there are three-leaf clovers, the three branches of the U.S. Federal Government and easy-to-balance three-legged stools.

In my quest for Serenity and Happiness, I discovered a three-pronged tool (no, it's not a fork) that I call my Triple Whammy of Love (and no it's not a way to seduce women in bars). My Triple Whammy of Love is a principle that helps me defeat the Misery Conspiracy at multiple levels. It's totally kickin'.

The Triple Whammy of Love comes from the Commandments put forth by Jesus when he was questioned by one of his followers. He said, "Love the Lord your God with all your heart, all your mind, and all your soul. And Love your neighbor as yourself." The Greek word for "Love" used here is *agape*, which means a Divine, unconditional Love, as opposed to a romantic (*eros*) or brotherly (*philio*) love.

My Triple Whammy of Love is pared down and broken out a little differently. Here's what I have:

- Love God unconditionally.
- Love each other unconditionally.
- Love yourself unconditionally.

Regardless of your religious tradition, it is essential to connect to our Spiritual Source, as I've said before. This means that we allow for the free flow of Love between ourselves and our Source. We extend love to God, not because God will feel offended if we don't, but because to do otherwise is to block ourselves off from the flow of Love back to us. Allowing the flow opens us up to the experience of Unity or Oneness with our Spiritual Source. This is the experience of Heaven or Bliss.

In the same vein, it's not enough just to Love someone else with the same amount of Love that we have for ourselves. People who Love themselves unconditionally naturally Love everyone else unconditionally. And people who withhold Love from others do so, in part, because they don't Love themselves very much. It's a fundamental principal of Spiritual Dynamics. We either allow for the free flow of Love to all others (not just the ones we think deserve Love) or we block ourselves off from the flow.

As we practice this Triple Whammy of Love principle, we return to our original state of Peace and Joy. Fear loses its foothold in our minds and can no longer block our experience of Heaven. As Jesus said, "The Kingdom of Heaven is at hand." It's in our minds. We need only to Love God, each other and ourselves unconditionally to experience it in this very moment. You don't even have to wait for your body to quit working. It's available whenever you are.

Whenever you get into crisis, pull out this tool and put ask yourself: Are you Loving and reaching out to the God of your understanding? Are you opening yourself up to the presence of the Divine in you? Are you honoring it? And are you open to seeing the Divine in everyone around you, regardless of how they are behaving? Make this three-fold principle your mantra, and it will always steer you towards Peace.

Chapter 35:
Placebos, Visualization and Black Feathers

Our minds are amazing things. Their capacity to create and love and understand and most of all, change, is phenomenal. But sometimes our minds need a little help, a temporary crutch to get us over the humps of our disbelief. These crutches are also sacred tools of the Spirit.

In the Disney classic, *Dumbo*, the young elephant with the enormous ears encounters a flock of crows who agree to teach him how to fly. As part of the lessons, the crows bestow upon Dumbo the Black Feather, a magical talisman that they give to all young crows learning to fly. To his amazement and delight, Dumbo finds that with the Black Feather grasped firmly in his trunk, he can indeed fly like a bird.

What the naïve, yet gifted, little elephant doesn't know is that he can already fly. He's just been asleep every time he's done it. All he needed in order to do it in his waking hours was a firm belief in his abilities. The crows had watched him do it in his sleep, which is why they gave him the Black Feather. There was nothing magical about the feather it all. But it served as a temporary device to help Dumbo establish his belief in himself.

So what does this animated classic, and specifically the story of the Black Feather, have to do with combating the Misery Conspiracy? Sometimes, in order to access the tremendous power of our mind, we occasionally need to use certain objects or circumstances. To further illustrate my point, let's take a look at the world of medicine.

It is common practice during the testing of new drugs to have a control group. The control group doesn't get to take the new drug. What they get is a placebo, which is just a sugar pill. However, the members of the control group don't know it's a placebo. They don't even know that they are in the control group. As far as they know, they're taking the new drug. The medical community designs blind studies this way to eliminate what's called the "placebo effect" from their results.

If the lab is testing a new drug to stop migraine headaches, for instance, they need to know if the drug is really having a positive effect. They give new drug to the test group and a placebo to the control group. If the test group has a 70% recovery rate (meaning the migraine goes away) but the control group has a significantly lower recovery rate (say 30%), then the drug must be having a positive effect.

What I find interesting isn't the 70% recovery rate of the test group. Don't get me wrong, I'm glad the drug works. What really fascinates me is the 30% recovery rate (or whatever it is) in the control group. Somehow, they managed to get rid of their migraine from the sheer belief that they were taking the drug. As a sufferer from migraines myself, I find that amazing!

In the field of sports psychology, athletes are encouraged to visualize themselves performing at levels greater than their personal best. In their minds, they see themselves hitting a home run or nailing a free throw or clearing the high bar. When they do this, their performances improve. When harnessing the power of belief, the mind can push us to greater accomplishments than we previously imagined.

We can harness this same power to free ourselves from the grip of the Misery Conspiracy. I can't tell you how many times I hear people say things like, "He made me angry," or "I can't get out of this depression," or "I'm trapped in a dead-end job."

I want to pound my forehead every time these words assault my ears. I want to shout at them, "No one can *make* you angry! You're not trapped in your depression or your job!" Not that shouting at these people, or even attempting to reason with them, would do any good.

These are limits that we put on ourselves, the same way that Dumbo was limiting his ability to fly. The Misery Conspiracy is always reminding us that we can't do this, or that we're stuck in that situation, or that someone else has control of our thoughts and emotions.

To break past these limits, we sometimes need an intermediary step. We need a temporary mental crutch on which to build our belief. We need our magical Black Feather to help lift us above the limits of the Misery Conspiracy. So long as it's only temporary, there is nothing wrong with that. Eventually, though, we have to learn to do it without the feather.

These Black Feathers come in the form of inspiring music, thought-provoking books and even religious rituals and objects. Theoretically, we have the potential to experience total Bliss right this instant. We can experience Oneness or Unity with God and each other. We can even manifest whatever we desire by simply willing it into being. At least, in theory!

It is only our disbelief, our lack of faith and understanding, that prevents us from doing these things. To move past these mental barriers, we use our Black Feathers. We listen to music that lifts our spirits. We read books like this one that remind us of who we are and what we are capable of doing. We practice various traditions as a symbolic way of teaching spiritual truths to our subconscious.

Eventually the human race will evolve to the point where we won't need the books or music or rituals to experience our Unity with God and each other. We won't need drugs to heal illness or injury. That's not really as far out as it may seem. Already, meditation and other spiritual tools are used to improve a patient's chances of combating cancer, HIV and other serious medical conditions. It is the natural inclination of our bodies and our minds to heal themselves.

When was the last time you had to cause your blood to clot? How is it that your body defends itself against deadly microbes every day? All doctors can do with a broken leg is set it and then let the body's natural process of healing take over. Amazing! Why shouldn't we believe that we will one day take that ability to a whole new level? What are we but energy and consciousness?

If you don't know how to be Happy in the face of chaotic situations, such as a divorce or getting fired or losing a loved one, don't panic. And don't resign yourself to misery! Open yourself to the possibility, and take what logical steps need to be taken to work through it. Read a book. Listen to some uplifting music. Go to a support group.

These are all Black Feathers to give you enough confidence to claim your own power. Pretty soon, you'll be flying without them.

Chapter 36:
Dusty Toolboxes and Hurricane Lists

The tools that I have shared with you in this section are powerful and can really help you defeat the Misery Conspiracy. There is one caveat: you actually have to use the tools. Knowing about the tools is good. Understanding how they work is great. But unless we put them to use, they are just a lot of great concepts. If you're tired of being miserable, it's not enough to say, "Oh yeah! I know how to handle that situation." You have to do something about the situation, even if it's just to say to yourself, "I'm willing to see this differently."

Between the time I got sober and the time I left my ex-husband Ray for good (third time was the charm), I still had a lot of drama in my life. I was still so newly sober that I didn't know how to handle situations when they got crazy or when life got so quiet that I would get caught up in my self-pity and alcoholic thinking. With the help of my friends in recovery and especially my sponsor, I learned about a lot of things I could do in those situations. But when the circumstances arose, I totally forgot about them and would get caught up in the drama.

My sponsor understood this dilemma. She sat down with me one Saturday afternoon and made me write out two lists. The first list was a Hurricane List, which included things to do when situations got out of control. The rules, according to my sponsor, were that if when life started turning into an emotional hurricane (e.g., Ray started raging or shaming), I had to do one of the activities on the list. And if after doing that, things were still chaotic, I had to continue doing items on the list until the "hurricane" was over.

The list included such things as:

- Remove yourself from the hurricane (situation)
- If necessary (i.e. you are in physical danger), call 911.
- Go to a meeting
- Call your sponsor or a friend from one of your meetings
- Read from the AA Big Book or similar material
- Pray
- Meditate
- Journal

The next was a Doldrums List, which was very similar to the Hurricane List, but was designed to get me out of my obsessive, negative thinking. It's called the Doldrums List because the Doldrums are a place in the ocean where there are few winds or currents. Before the advent of the steam engine, this was a dangerous place to be because you could be stranded there for weeks, just baking in the sun as your supplies of food and fresh water vanished. People get "cabin fever".

I have learned that if I'm not careful, I can easily get into a similar mindset if I'm not properly nourishing my spirit on a regular basis. This list still comes in handy today. It includes the following:

- Be willing to see things differently.
- Go to a meeting.
- Call your sponsor or a friend.
- Read the AA Big Book or similar material
- Pray
- Meditate
- Go climb a mountain (there are a lot of them in Phoenix)
- Find someone in need and help them.

As with the Hurricane List, the rule is that I have do pick something on this list and do it. And if I still feel in the Doldrums afterwards, I have to pick something else and keep doing things on the list until my thinking changes.

I always kept these lists with me; either in my purse or in my AA Big Book. As I used them, my recovery process skyrocketed. When things got crazy or I got crazy, I would pull out my list and start doing the recommended activities until life started to settle down. Sometimes I had to do three or four items on the list before I could quit. A few times I went through everything on the list and had to repeat a few before the hurricane passed or I could feel that spiritual push from my Higher Power.

Even now, I keep these lists handy because there is a strong temptation to think about the tools in my Spiritual Toolbox, but to not actually implement any of them. My addictive thought process (what I call my *crazies*) tries to tell me, "You don't want to call anyone. They're busy with their own lives. You won't find anything uplifting in the AA Big Book. You've already read it a dozen times." That's why the rules are so important. I *know* that I have to pick something on the list and *do* it, not just think about it. And I have to keep picking stuff to do until the *crazies* go away.

If you are tired of being miserable, it's time to sit down and make a couple of lists yourself. Feel free to borrow from mine and add your own activities. It helps to keep a list of names and phone numbers of people to call with that list, so that you can't say, "Oh, I don't know anyone's number." You just start at the top of the list and keep calling until you reach someone (voice mail doesn't count), and after talking with them, you feel better. If you're in recovery, you will also want a comprehensive list of meetings, so that even if it's 9:00 on a Sunday night, you will know where you can go. A lot of these meetings are listed online, but you don't want to go searching when you're in the hurricane.

Don't let dust collect on your Spiritual Toolbox. The tools presented in this section can only help you fight the Misery Conspiracy if you use them. They are useless otherwise. You have a right to be Happy. To claim that right, you have to exercise it. And exercise means you have to get off you derriere and do something. It's worth it!

Section Four:
Breaking Out Of
Maximum Security Misery

Chapter 37:
Finding Peace through Forgiveness

Forgiveness is such an amazing, profound, yet misunderstood, spiritual tool that I felt the need to devote an entire section to it. Forgiveness is the tool that frees us from the burden of the past. We all carry the weight of past hurts, traumas and loss. We have been led to believe by the Misery Conspiracy that we are doomed to drag these burdens with us forever; that we have been permanently scarred, and will never be whole again. To that I say, "What a load of crap!"

What someone did to us in the past may have been painful, but to hold onto it in the present and continuously twist it in our minds only prolongs the pain. We keep looking to understand why we were victimized, not realizing that we are victimizing *ourselves* in our search for answers where there are none. The solution is to let ourselves off the hook by letting go of the trauma itself.

To start off this section, I want to share with you a speech I gave at the women's retreat that I mentioned earlier in the book. Despite all of the chaos that went on as I gave my presentation, I believe that this exercise has great value in teaching us how to free both ourselves and our perpetrators (yes, even them) from the Misery Conspiracy's weapon of resentment.

Here is my presentation in its entirety (minus the crackle of the bonfire, the sweet scent of the juniper trees, and the night sky jam-packed with stars):

~~~~~~~~~~~~~~~~~~~~~~~~~~~~~

The name of this session of Emergence, this retreat, is Light. We have just experienced a beautiful day with a beautiful blue sky. Now we are sitting here in the dark, and yet we know that the sun continues to shine. It is just obscured by the Earth.

Light is Spirit. Light is Love. Light is Peace of Mind. But so much of the time we sit here in the dark. The Divine Light still shines, but it is obscured by our resentments, our judgments, and all other forms of our fear-based thinking. As a result, our minds are filled with anger, fear, regret, and despair. To find our way back to the Light, we need only remove the blocks to our awareness of Love's presence, and the way to do it is through Forgiveness.

In Lesson 121 of the Workbook for *A Course in Miracles*, it says, "Forgiveness is the key to Happiness. Here is the answer to your search for Peace. Here is the key to meaning in a world that seems to make no sense."

Marianne Williamson said, "Forgiveness is the key to inner Peace because it is the mental technique by which our thoughts are transformed from fear to Love." She says, "The practice of Forgiveness is our most important contribution to the healing of the world. Angry people cannot create a peaceful planet."

When Jesus told us to Forgive others as we are Forgiven, he wasn't just telling us to be nice. He was explaining a crucial universal principle. By letting go of our judgments of others, we naturally release ourselves.

Tonight, we sit in darkness. And yet within us, the Light continues to shine as brilliantly as ever. This evening, I share with you the Sacred Key that will open the door for you to return to your natural state of Love and to a Peace beyond all understanding. We do this not for anyone else's sake. We do this for ourselves.

Before I begin this exercise, it is important that you understand what Forgiveness is. Forgiveness doesn't mean that what someone did to you was acceptable. Forgiveness is the recognition that what we thought someone did to us has no permanent effect.
~~~~~~~~~~~~~~~~~~~~~~~~~~~~~

It means we are willing to see that the experiences of the past now exist only in our minds. Forgiveness is the letting go of everything that is not Love. By letting go of our emotional and spiritual attachment to negative past experiences, we are freeing *ourselves*. We are returning to the Light.

I want you to close your eyes and think of someone you do not like. It could be someone that you absolutely despise or someone that you simply don't enjoy spending time with. The form of your anger or dislike isn't important. You probably already have someone in mind. This person will do for our exercise.

Allow yourself to feel the tightness and the weight that your resentments towards this person cause. It feels like a burden on your chest. It shortens your breath. It makes your forehead feel tight. It ties your stomach in knots. Is this Peace? No! Is this what you want? No!

Now let us remember that we are expressions of our Divine Creator. We are Light and Love and Peace. And just as we have temporarily blocked our Light, the person that we have in our mind has done the same thing. Underneath all of their bitterness, violence, apathy, cruelty and anger is the same Child of God, the same capacity of unconditional Love. It is deeply hidden but it is there. And now we become willing to see it in our minds.

We start to see a small point of Light appearing from within our image of this person. We watch as this small point of golden Light begins to grow, slowly encompassing our entire vision of their body. We realize that they are not their actions. They are not their egos. They are not their fear-based belief systems. We realize that underneath all of the masks of fear is our spiritual brother or sister.

And so we tell this person, either silently or aloud, "I want to be at Peace. I no longer desire to be burdened by my resentments towards you. I no longer want to be burdened by my anger. Therefore, I now choose to Forgive you for everything I thought you did to me. I release you now with Love forever."

We now let go of our attachment to their guilt and allow our Divine Light to merge with theirs and allow our unconditional

Love to flow through them. By doing so, the heaviness that we felt in our hearts just a little while ago begins to lift. Our chests feel light and free. Our foreheads are relaxed. We are no longer burdened by our judgment of them. We let the darkness lift and allow our Divine Light to merge with theirs. We begin to feel a profound Peace.

Now open your eyes and allow yourself to see in every woman here, including yourself, the same Divine Presence that you saw in your former enemy. Remember that when we withhold Love from anyone for any reason, we withhold it from everybody, including ourselves.

So as we continue the retreat, as we go to sleep tonight, and as we return home tomorrow, let us try to make a regular practice of letting go of everything that is not Love. Let us take time every morning and evening to allow ourselves to see the Divine Presence in everyone, and in doing so, we will see it in ourselves.

Chapter 38:
Gentle Vigilance

Many years ago, I took karate lessons at a little dojo in Glendale, Arizona. The sensei was this short fellow from Okinawa whose grasp of English was only slightly better than my grasp of nuclear physics. It was like something right out of Karate Kid II, only without the wax-on, wax off exercises. It was *intense*!

At the time, I was in decent shape for a gal in her mid-30s, but I had the flexibility of a rock. I also had no clue about the rules of protocol in the dojo. I got busted for every imaginable offense: folding my hands behind me as I stood at attention, exposing the bottoms of my feet in the general direction of the sensei, and not being able to understand the sensei's Japanenglish commands! And the shaming techniques for such infractions would rival even my Jewish-Catholic family's guilt trips. I quit after about four weeks.

Learning new skills can be tough, especially in a non-supportive environment. How we approach the task and ourselves can mean the difference between mastery and misery. When we accept nothing less than a perfect performance with minimal practice, we have a seriously flawed expectation on our hands. And as we say in AA, expectations are pre-meditated resentments.

Too many of us beat ourselves up over minor, stupid stuff! Admit it! You do it all the time! You chastise yourself for that typo in your email to the boss that made it sound like he was an idiot. You curse yourself for showing up to work in your jeans because you thought it was Friday (and spent two hours driving home, changing into business attire, and driving back to work). You obsess about that piece of cake you ate at the office party. And let's not forget about the check you forgot to record in your register that resulted in a cascade of NSFs and bank fees. Ouch!

Makes you wince, doesn't it? Thought so! And why? Shaming yourself only reinforces the lies of the Misery Conspiracy. *I'm stupid. I'm lazy. I'm fat. I'm irresponsible.* It's time to let ourselves off the hook. One way to do this is with gentle vigilance.

Gentle vigilance recognizes that mistakes, shortcomings and character flaws are a natural part of the learning process. It says, "Yes, you're going to screw up. But everybody screws up, so just chill!"

We all know that meditation is a keystone to any serious spiritual practice, right? It's that essential rebooting for our soul. When we don't do meditate on a regular basis, our thinking starts to get funky, and no one wants to be around us, not even our dog.

So being the enlightened guru that I am, naturally I put in 30 minutes sitting time every morning *minimum*! Yeah, right! I wish I did. My life would run a lot smoother if I did. When I do take the time to commune with the Universe, I am more Peaceful, joyful, and stable. And people like being around me! What a surprise!

A lot of people have difficulties making meditation a priority in their lives. There always seems to be some other urgent task to take care of, and THEN they'll meditate. Something always seems to come up. *Oh, today, I have to take the car into the shop. Tomorrow? Oh, I have to pick up the dry cleaning. Then it's an early morning milk run or a 7:30 a.m. department meeting or whatever.*

When we finally manage to sit down, our minds act like rabid hamsters spinning round and round. We try focusing on our breath and our mind focuses on that persistent sniffle we've had all day. We try to visualize rising out of our bodies and we start questioning whether or not we are visualizing it right. *What exactly am I seeing that's rising out of my body? Did I open my chakras in the right order? What does the orange one represent again?* And suddenly we realize we're thinking again and we open our eyes and say, "Screw it! I can't do this!" But you can do it. It just takes practice and gentle vigilance.

Gentle vigilance means that while we are continuous in our efforts to meditate, we don't beat ourselves up when we don't do it "just right." What sense does it make to get upset about how we do something that's supposed to make us more Peaceful? So what if we don't do the way someone told us to do it? If we just allow ourselves to make the mistakes everybody makes and learn from them, we'll find our own way to do it. That's what gentle vigilance is about.

Gentle vigilance lets go of expectations. We accept the situation for what it is. When you meditate, your mind is naturally going to wander at first. When it does, become aware of it, release the thought and gently bring your mind back to center. No shame! Just acceptance. With gentle vigilance, you simply start again. Simple, huh?

In recovery, we focus on progress rather than perfection. We understand that it is better to learn from our mistakes than to obsess about them. We also know that our mistakes don't define who we are. They have no bearing on our worth. Their sole purpose is to show us where we need to change.

Gentle vigilance works for many more situations than just our meditation practice. We can use it to improve our relationship with food, if that's an issue for us. With gentle vigilance, we don't beat ourselves up over eating a piece of cake at an office birthday party. Instead, we acknowledge the consequences of our choices and then choose differently in the future.

Gentle vigilance works for any situation that we are struggling with or any new skill that we are learning. If I had applied gentle vigilance to my karate lessons, perhaps I would still be doing it. Perhaps I would have moved beyond the white belt. Perhaps I would be able to touch my toes. Or not.

Chapter 39:
Pitch Blue

Back when I was a girl with a torch designing jewelry, a visual artist friend of mine told me something interesting. Black ink isn't really black. It's more of a blue-black; a pitch blue, if you will. Okay, that probably doesn't sound that interesting to you. "Black ink isn't blue. Big woop!" But sometimes it's these silly little things that give me a new perspective on something more dramatic.

I find this an interesting fact; that which appears to be without light, without color, does, in fact, hold a faint glimmer of color or light, like the depths of the ocean where only fish and remote alien civilizations live (okay, that was just a movie).

Before Bill W. and Dr. Bob started Alcoholics Anonymous nearly a century ago, alcoholics were considered hopeless. Even the most advanced psychotherapy at the time had little effect in keeping an alcoholic from relapsing.

Even today, there are people we classify as unredeemable: pedophiles, sociopathic murderers, and politicians (they seem physiologically incapable of telling the truth in spite of overwhelming evidence). But if a handful of drunks could figure out how to stay sober (even after psychologists had written them off), perhaps there is yet hope for the others.

"Their hearts are black," we claim. "They don't deserve to live because of the harm they've caused." But at the risk of sounding like a bleeding heart liberal (okay, I am one), I invite you to take another look and consider new possibilities.

As I mentioned in the previous chapter, we are not our mistakes. And the people that we see as unredeemable aren't their mistakes either. Yeah, I know. That's a hard one to swallow. And I'm not saying that they shouldn't be held responsible for their actions. Boundaries on behavior have to set.

But it is important that we remember who we are: the innocent Children of the Divine, who believed that we were something else. Maybe we came into this world with bad wiring or we experienced a trauma that scrambled our brains. So we see ourselves as separate from the Universe. We think we're guilty and unlovable.

To cope with these lies of the Misery Conspiracy, to fend off attacks that we fear are coming, we have built thick walls around our imaginary "little selves", a.k.a. our egos. We wear armor so thick that no glimmer of Light can peek through. And we have worn it so long, that even we have forgotten that our true nature still exists.

If this is true for you and me (and it is), then it is also true for those we see as unredeemable. Yeah, we can't see any hint of humanity in their nature; no Compassion, no contrition, no sense of morality. They certainly don't seem to be suffering from their stone cold natures. They may even seem gleeful about the harm they inflict on others. But underneath all of the armor of the ego, there remains what can be hidden, but never destroyed: the innocent Child of Universe.

"Innocent?" you say? "After what they did to me, to my child, to those innocent civilians?" And to that I calmly answer, "Yes." Sure, what they did was horrible, sadistic, and cruel. But like the rest of us, they were operating based on a seriously flawed belief system. That's what the Misery Conspiracy does to people.

I don't propose putting "pink paint" on the situation, to quote Marianne Williamson. I'm certainly not suggesting that such people should be allowed to continue their harmful behavior. But executing them doesn't solve the problem. It doesn't heal the hurt or close the wound. Only Forgiveness can do that. It doesn't change the nature of their broken Spirit. As the Children of God, they are Spirit, and if we kill their bodies, they will show up in another form and we will have to deal with them again.

Just locking them up doesn't solve the problem unless we, as a society, take the time to undo the hate and hurt and fear. It is only when we make a sustained and permanent effort to heal these wounds (and this could take millennia or longer) that the problem will be undone. If the quick fixes of execution and imprisonment, we would have seen an improvement a long time ago. It's time to let the real healing begin.

Forgiveness and Compassion are not the naïve way out that the Misery Conspiracy would suggest they are. In fact, it takes a greater commitment than what we currently give to these people. But there is no way around it. How long we take before we are willing to let go of our hatred for these "black-hearted" people is up to us, but it is the only solution.

So the next time you feel anger towards someone, remember that their hearts aren't black. They are just very, very dark pitch blue. Be willing to see them differently. Be willing to let go of everything but love. Be willing to consider a new approach to responding to the "unredeemable".

Chapter 40:
The Prodigal Son Revisited

Recently, I was recalling Jesus' parable of the Prodigal Son. This is a classic story that speaks to the issue of Divine Forgiveness. Despite its popularity, it amazes me how many people, especially Christians, totally ignore the lessons it teaches. They still portray God as this angry, vengeful deity, demanding a blood sacrifice to appease his wounded ego. Talk about a dark, twisted vision of the Divine!

Oh, if only we would just pay attention to the lessons right under our noses! My point is that Jesus' parable paints a different picture and shows us the proper place for Forgiveness.

The point of the parable was that the father had welcomed his son home in spite of all of the mistakes that the son had made. The son had squandered his share of his father's inheritance, and yet the father welcomed him home with open arms. The father didn't care about the money, or his son's foolish, decadent behavior. He was simply glad to have his son home safe again. Wouldn't you? Also, the father didn't wait for the son to come home to Forgive him. He forgave him the moment he left home.

Clearly the father in the story represents God. It teaches that God isn't obsessed with "sin" the way so many of us are. We have this whole Goth drama going on, when God only wants us Home, safe in the reality of His Love. And isn't that what we want, too?

Unfortunately, the Misery Conspiracy offers up a very different view of God. If the Misery Conspiracy were to rewrite the parable, the father would have had to kill the good son (the one that never left) in order to "atone" for the sins of the prodigal son. Doesn't make a lot of sense, does it?

It is a common misconception that God holds a grudge against his children for their sins, and that only Jesus' blood on the cross could atone for that sin. What kind of father demands the shedding of blood to pay for the mistakes of a child? When we really look at it, this is a very bloodthirsty misrepresentation of God. It is not the portrait of God that Jesus and many other enlightened masters teach us.

The word used in the Greek translation of the Bible to describe God's Love for humanity is *agape*, which means unconditional Love. If God's Love is unconditional, then there is *nothing* that we could ever do that would make God withhold His Love. We can close ourselves off from our experience of His Love, but we cannot make God stop loving us.

Some people would have you think that just by being born, we are corrupted with "original sin" and are outside God's Love right out of the gate. What really breaks my heart is that people actually believe that lie. They really believe that they are somehow unlovable, and then project that guilt on those around them. How sad is that? Too often we become tangled in our own fear and hatred, teaching that God is bloodthirsty and unforgiving. This is not what Jesus taught.

I encourage you to actually read the teachings of Jesus, whether or not you are a Christian. See how he treats people and then follow his example. Remember that the loving father welcomes his son home with open arms, not at the point of a sword.

Jesus is a guide, one who knows the way Home. "I am the way, the truth and the life," means that he came to demonstrate what we need to do to return to a Peace that passes all understanding. He told us to Love God, to Love each other, and to Love ourselves. He taught us to stop judging each other. He repeatedly demonstrated Compassion to those the priesthood considered unworthy of Compassion.

The next time someone tries to tell you that God's going to send you to Hell, remind them of this parable. Then open your heart to all of the "prodigal sons" in your life, rather than being resentful like the son who never left. And like the father, we don't need to wait for someone to apologize and make amends for us to Forgive them. We can go ahead and Forgive them now, paving the way for them to come Home.

Chapter 41:
Forgiving Our Attackers

Some of us were abused and molested as children. It is so traumatic to endure such predatory behavior when we are so young. It creates wounds that stay with us for a long time. We learn to wear the badge of "victim", either proudly or privately. But it is this very identity that continues the trauma. Forgiving our perpetrators, as undeserved as it may seem, is the key to our freedom.

Once my friend, Ellie found herself in a very humiliating situation. Wanting to do something bold to celebrate her birthday, she agreed to pose for a nude drawing. The "artist" drawing the portrait is a celebrated architect, now in his 70's or 80's. The problem came when this architect/artist started displaying a complete lack of professionalism, leading to behaviors common in sexual predators.

While in the middle of drawing one of the nudes, he asked Ellie if he could lick her nipples. She was offended, but politely told him "no." Then, after finishing the portrait, he licked his finger and rubbed the breasts in the drawing, saying "Mmmm...pretty nipples." Then when he finally showed her the finished portraits, he pointed out to her that in a few of the drawings, he intentionally drew Ellie with a child's face and no pubic hair, suggesting an attraction to young girls.

The artist's sexually aggressive behavior upset Ellie, triggering memories of when her grandfather molested her when she was young. She felt humiliated and emotionally violated. Her previous fears and distrust of older men were confirmed once again. She was convinced that she would never be able to Forgive this man for his violations of her trust.

Having survived being raped myself, I can appreciate her response. It is important for her to feel her feelings and to work through them. But as *A Course in Miracles* teaches, the situation can be used either to strengthen fear or to overcome it and expand Love instead. It is up to us to decide which purpose the situation serves.

My friend, Ellie, has a right to feel angry and hurt. But maybe this situation came up so that she can finally get over the issue of her grandfather's abuse. This does not justify the predatory actions of either her grandfather or the artist. In fact, it has nothing to do with them. It has everything to do with her rising above vulnerability, so that she can find Peace again.

Fear, regardless of form (depression, anger, violence, etc.), is always a result of judging others or ourselves as unworthy of Love. It is a block to Love that we have created. Forgiveness is simply removing that block to Love. It is the recognition that when we judge people, we feel miserable. It is also the recognition that we are not bodies and we are not what our bodies do or say. We are Spirit, the sacred Children of God, who are lost in an illusionary nightmare that we made.

When we have been violated and are suffering, we must find a way to free ourselves from the loveless thought patterns in our minds. To do this, we must Forgive our attacker(s) by letting go of our loveless thoughts about them. It often takes a conscious effort to do so, asking God for a miracle to change our thoughts from anger and upset to Peace and Love.

This doesn't mean we let people walk all over us. We can honor our boundaries at the same time that we demonstrate Love. We can put an end to inappropriate behavior towards us without resenting or attacking the person who is acting out. When we do, we are no longer victims, but powerful beings transforming the planet.

Chapter 42:
Who's Your Enemy?

A prolonged conflict leaves many wounds on both sides. In a marriage, it creates a myriad of trigger issues, any one of which can be used to launch into a tirade of shame and guilt against the other person. When I was married to my ex-husband, my panel of hot buttons was as extensive as the cockpit of the space shuttle Discovery. Fortunately, I have managed to remove and/or dismantle most of these buttons (mine, not the shuttle's).

In the case of a war, such as the one between the Israeli and Palestinian people, a prolonged conflict leaves thousands dead. Those who survive make it their mission to cling to their losses, keeping the wounds fresh in their minds and vowing complete and ultimate destruction of the enemy. Despite what the Misery Conspiracy tells us, this will not bring us inner Peace any more than it brings outer peace.

When Palestinian leader Yasser Arafat died, many hoped it might serve as a turning point for the conflict. Some celebrated his death, figuratively dancing on his grave. Others grieved his passing. In the media, a long parade of pundits described him as everything from the last hope for peace to a corrupt leader to the devil incarnate. Who he was seemed entirely to depend on the personal agenda of the person you asked. Interesting!

On the level of form, this conflict between the Palestinians and the Israelis seems very confusing and convoluted. There are so many historical claims for both sides. Deciding who the land belongs to has everything to do with where you put your finger in time. Is it the Palestinians, the Israelis, the Greeks, the Romans, the French, the Babylonians, the Assyrians, the Persians, the Egyptians or the Turks? All at one time or another have controlled this tiny strip of land that has been painted with too much blood and tears.

Too many innocent civilians have been killed by both sides of the current conflict. Too many violations of trust have been perpetrated by both sides. And too many people have refused to look at the suffering of "the other." Between the suicide bombers and the overly aggressive retaliations, the pledges of eternal jihad, and the building of Sharon's wall across Palestinian farms, there seems to be no solution in sight.

But on a much deeper level, on the level of content, the solution is simple. From this perspective, there are only two choices: Love and fear. For thousands of years, fear has reigned. Fear in the form of suicide bombers, military actions, 6-Day Wars, the murder of Olympic athletes, etc. The forms of fear are endless and they offer no hope for peace. Only when we turn away from fear and consider the alternative (Love) can hope be found. Any roadmap to peace must revolve around Love.

There are so many things that people point to as reasons *not* to Forgive their "enemy." To a one, every one of these reasons center on something from the past. But the past, as even Einstein and Carl Sagan pointed out, exists only in our minds. The past is an illusion. The future is also an illusion. Time itself is an illusion. We are divine, eternal beings. Forgiveness is simply the letting go of illusions.

Despite the hopes of some, the death of Chairman Arafat changed nothing in the Palestine-Israel conflict. The ideals and beliefs that he held to, whatever they may have been, were surely shared by others in Palestine, and perhaps in Israel too. Whether he was a visionary of peace or a slippery politician or a crazed warmongerer, he is not the only one to have had this approach.

Meanwhile, the ego drama that is the Palestinian-Israeli conflict continues on. The fighting won't stop just because a heart stopped beating. So if we are tired of suicide bombers and overly aggressive Israeli actions, we have to change this from a world of resentments to a world of Love. We have to change the dream from a nightmare to a Peaceful dream.

A Course in Miracles tells us that if we want to change the world we see, we have to change our minds about it. We have to let go of our attachment to judgment, fear, and anger. We must be willing to forgive even the most heinous of illusionary crimes.

A real test of our willingness to forgive is when our so-called enemies are praised and given accolades. Despite being raised Catholic (or maybe because of it), I never had a great affinity for Pope John Paul II. His views on a variety of issues conflicted with mine, making it difficult for me to see him as anything but a maintainer of the status quo for medieval attitudes.

When he died, the news networks were a-flurry with reports of his death, showcasing his funeral and speculating on who his successor would be. That's what the news media does, after all. But what really got to me was all of the stories about what a caring and spiritually-minded man he was. That was a hot button for me that had not yet been dismantled.

At the time, my negative thought process launched into a tirade about his unwillingness to *even discuss* the issue of women clergy and his long-standing opposition to birth control, not to mention the Church's atrocious record of covering up cases of child-molesting priests. It's embarrassing to admit. A man was dead, and all I could focus on was what *he did wrong* in life. I wanted to sing, "Ding! Ding! The Pope is dead!" I wanted to dance on the grave of my "enemy".

There is a word for this in German. *Schadenfreude* is the celebration of the suffering or misfortune of others. When you're driving down the highway and the guy who cut you off ten minutes ago gets pulled over by the police for speeding, and you laugh at his misfortune, that's *schadenfreude*. When a politician you hate gets booted out of office, and you celebrate, that's *schadenfreude*. When Ms. Schwartz' yippy schnauzer from next door falls down the trash chute and you not only ignore it, but cheer it, that's *schadenfreude*.

In the case of my rejoicing the Pontiff's passing, it was *schadenfreude* and it was wrong. Fortunately, I was quickly reminded by a friend that regardless of my opinion of him (which was so one-sidedly inaccurate as to be almost funny), celebrating his death wasn't a very enlightened thing to do.

It's embarrassing to teach about Forgiveness, only to get busted in the act of not forgiving. Yet I am grateful for the opportunity to be reminded of this essential lesson yet again. After all, this *is* how we learn – by making the same stupid mistakes over and over again. I learn a lot of things this way.

Pope John Paul II was not a perfect man. And while I never saw it personally, I am sure that, in most situations, he was a very caring, compassionate man. Certainly his work in Poland for Polish solidarity is commendable. And if *he* could forgive the man who attempted to assassinate him, who was I not to let go of my resentments towards *him*?

If I am to find Peace, I must let go of everything that is not Love. If I am to experience Heaven, I must be willing to see the presence of God in everyone, including a man that the Misery Conspiracy tells me was misogynistic, homophobic, and possibly corrupt. And so I wish him only Love, Peace and Healing in his continuing journey, wherever it takes him. I honor the things he did that were Loving, and let go of the rest.

Who are your enemies? Are there certain politicians who make your blood boil every time their faces appear on the news? Are there people you work with who get praised for their inferior work while your efforts are totally ignored? It's so unfair, isn't it? Well, get over it! Forget about fairness. It's time to let it go of your resentments. It's not affecting them, but it's eating you alive. *Schadenfreude* will destroy ya! The best way to vanquish your enemies is by turning them into friends.

Chapter 43:
Coping with Unrequited Compassion

My friend Dave doesn't trust people. He's an awesome guy in all other aspects. He's smart and creative and passionate. He is also very respectful of women, almost to the point of being protective of them. If I were straight and single, he would rank high on my list of guys worth dating. But as sweet and as charming as he is, he just doesn't trust people. Not a one! From his perspective, most people are jerks and will rip you off at the first opportunity.

I once asked him why he had such a negative view of people. In reply, he related an experience he had had with a former roommate. It seems that when his buddy Joey was down on his luck, Dave asked his parents to allow his friend to stay with them until he could get back on his feet. His parents agreed, trusting Dave's judgment of character.

After several months of living rent-free, however, Joey disappeared with thousands of dollars' worth of his hosts' belongings. As it turns out, Joey had a bit of a drug problem that demanded large amounts of cash on a regular basis. While Dave's parents took the loss in stride, Dave was devastated.

Coming from a traditional Japanese family, Dave felt that he had lost face with his father. His Compassion for a friend in need had been met with a slap in the face. And his parents had paid the price for his poor judgment. He felt betrayed, ashamed, and bitter, refusing to offer such generosity to anyone again.

A lot of people are reluctant to be compassionate when past efforts to help others have been met with ingratitude, apathy, betrayal, or hostility. Who wouldn't be reluctant? Why help people out if our efforts are unappreciated? In short, unrequited compassion sucks!

But here's the thing – there is no such thing as unrequited compassion. No act of love or compassion is ever wasted. It's just that some people are so shut down that no light can be seen from within. Years of trauma, abuse, and neglect have pushed people to build such thick armor around their hearts, that we simply can't see an effect.

But what's going on is that every act of compassion softens that armor just a little bit. A single act of kindness isn't likely to turn that around overnight, but each one moves that person closer to the point of opening up.

In my recovery from addiction and depression, I have heard hundreds, if not thousands, of stories from people who were shut down at one point in their lives. Before getting clean, they were just mean drunks, deceitful drug addicts, and even merciless criminals. Acts of Compassion from others were met with denial and retaliation. Every message of "I care about you" faced a history of messages from people who didn't care. It took most of us a long time before we finally hit bottom.

In the safety of support and recovery groups, Acceptance and Forgiveness were at last able to reach our hearts and heal our spirits. And here, the benefits of those previous acts of generosity (that at one time seemed unrequited) were finally appreciated and eventually paid back or even paid forward to others.

This doesn't mean that we have to become doormats or subject ourselves to people we know are, at least temporarily, untrustworthy. I am an advocate of using discernment to make the best use of generosity. Enabling addictive or antisocial behavior isn't noble. But neither should we close our hearts to those in need.

Rather, we should give in ways that honor both giver and receiver. If that means giving materially, fine. It can also mean we simply spend time with someone or just say a heartfelt prayer for their healing.

No act of generosity is wasted. And even in cases where the person in need is unable to respond in a positive way, no Compassion is really unrequited. At worst, it is delayed.

Chapter 44:
Who Will Teach Them?

I spoke earlier about how forgiveness isn't about letting someone else off the hook. The purpose of forgiveness – that is, letting go of our resentments and judgments – is to let ourselves off the hook. In a way, forgiveness is the spiritual equivalent of taking a dump after being constipated for years. It takes some effort. It feels uncomfortable at first. But when it's done, WHEW! What a relief! Okay, I admit it's kind of an icky parallel, but you get the point!

When we can finally free ourselves from the burden of our past hurts, it changes how we see the world. But if we really want to change the world we live in, we have to take the next step. We must participate in the healing of those we feel have harmed us. Just think of it as the clean-up after the dump! Okay, no more crap spirituality! I promise.

Let's talk criminal justice! I find it odd that most prison systems are operated by the local or state Department of *Corrections*. What kind of *correcting* is going on exactly? Is anyone (other than volunteers from a local church) taking the time to help inmates overcome the dysfunctional thought processes and belief systems that lead them to commit their very special crimes? Is anyone from the Department of Corrections helping the inmates *correct* their misperceptions and combat the lies of the Misery Conspiracy? Maybe we should just rename them "Departments of Incarceration".

We complain about the high recidivism rates of violent criminals and how it costs so much money to build more and more prisons. In Maricopa County, Arizona, Sheriff Joe Arpaio (long claimed to be the "toughest sheriff in America") puts inmates in what he calls Tent City. And if living in a tent in the Sonoran Desert isn't tough enough (with summer temps reaching 120º F), inmates get green baloney sandwiches for lunch and dinner and are forced to wear pink boxer shorts (I used to have a pair, but it's not what you think). They are not allowed access to porn or T.V. Sheriff Joe has been creative in the ways that he denies *luxuries* to his prisoners.

But for all their creativity, have any of these measures reduced the crime rates in Phoenix? Did the gangbangers and the meth dealers and the child-molesters and the rapists change their ways or move out of state? Would have been nice, but no! They're still here. Have these restrictions reduced the number of repeat offenders? Sadly, no! So if punishing the criminals isn't correcting their behavior, then what are our options? How do does the Department of Corrections get them to change? The answer is that they can't.

Don't get me wrong! I'm grateful that they take criminals off the street, if only for a little while. And I'm not criticizing the prison system for their attempts to handle a difficult and growing problem. At best, though, all the prison systems can do is attempt to contain the problem. They aren't equipped to solve it.

But what is the problem? Why do some people choose to violate the laws? What is it that makes them think that committing a crime is their best option? It has to do with how they see themselves and the world around them. When they seem themselves as powerless and/or worthless, struggling in a world that doesn't give a whit whether they live or die, they stop caring about following the rules. When following the rules won't get you what you want, then the rules get chucked out the window.

When we live in a society that blindly follows the Misery Conspiracy, where some people are valued and others discarded, crime is an inevitability. When we are constantly bombarded with commercial messages telling us that we are not enough as we are, then people will go to any length to attain whatever they think will make them enough. Why else would someone get into a brawl over buying a video game player on the day after Thanksgiving?

During their 2004 presidential campaigns, both Senator Kerry and President Bush announced that one of their goals was to hunt down the "terrorists" and kill them. Seeing the "evildoers" of the world get punished and suffer for their crimes may appeal to our sense of justice, but the truth is, it really doesn't solve the problem. Punishment for the purpose of causing suffering only perpetuates the Misery Conspiracy.

If we hate our enemies, who will teach them Love? If someone acts mean towards you, who does it help to act mean back to them? Look at the conflicts between Ireland and England and the conflicts between Israel and Palestine. It's the Hatfields and the McCoys all over again, only on a larger scale. Nobody even remembers who insulted whom first. They just know that more of "them" have to suffer and die. And so the killing continues and escalates until enough people realize that killing is not solving the problem.

If we want to reduce crime in our neighborhood, we have to make it a point to treat everyone that we meet with Love, Compassion and respect. We have to let people merge in front of us in traffic. We have to thank the cashier at the local burger joint for taking our order, even if he made a mistake. We need to smile at people, including those who make us nervous or who look like they just got release from prison (look for the pink boxers).

People act out in unloving ways because they feel unloved and unlovable. If we change their perception of themselves, if we show them that they are loved and lovable, they will no longer feel the need to act out. This is just as true for terrorists as it is for drunk drivers, as true for child molesters as it is for grumpy customer service reps.

The next time you feel the urge to hate someone, the next time you get upset at someone for something they said or did, remember that they are doing it from a place of lovelessness. Then, remind them through your actions, words, and most of all your thoughts, that they are loved and are lovable. If we don't teach them Love, who will?

Section Five:
Finding Peace
Amidst The Garbage

Chapter 45:
The Tragedy of the Plaster Buddha

For our honeymoon many years ago, Eileen and I went to Thailand for two weeks. It was an experience that I treasure to this day. The people there are so amazingly friendly and are even willing to try and speak English, even if what comes out isn't English.

I was also in love with the wide variety of foods I had never seen. On our first morning there, the hotel brought us a bowl of fresh fruit. Neither of us recognized any of the fruits in the bowl. It was an adventure to figure out how to eat each one, including what parts are edible and how to get at them. I must say that the rambutans, which resemble little red Koosh balls, were the most unusual and the tastiest.

In scouring the tourist guides before the trip, I learned about a remarkable event that occurred 50 years ago in the northern part of the country. A group of explorers had discovered an ancient Buddhist temple that had long been abandoned. Within this temple they found a 10-foot tall Buddha statue made of plaster.

The explorers decided to relocate it to a wat (Buddhist temple) closer to Bangkok so that more people could see it. Engineers were called out to handle the move. They estimated the weight of the statue, based on its size and the average weight of plaster. A crane was then used to lift it up and put it on a truck to transport it. But as the statue was being lifted, tragedy struck! The cable snapped, sending the plaster statue crashing to the ground and causing a huge crack along one side. The workers rushed in to see the extent of the damage. What they found amazed them.

Through the cracked plaster they discovered the reason the cable snapped. The statue wasn't really made of plaster. It was only *covered* in plaster. Underneath, they found a 10-foot tall Buddha made of pure gold and weighing an estimated 5 tons! What they had originally thought was a mere artifact turned out to be a priceless treasure.

Further research later revealed that, 500 years before, the Buddhist monks who lived there had covered it with plaster to hide it from a marauding army. Unfortunately, the monks never returned and the secret was forgotten until the statue was dropped and the plaster cracked.

From this story, I have learned two significant lessons. The first is that we think we're cheap plaster, but we're really a priceless treasure. We look at our bodies and our bank accounts and our job descriptions and our addictions and think that's who we are. We have totally lost touch with our true nature, our deeper spiritual Self. And that's where the treasure is. That's where the Happiness and Joy and Serenity is. That's the good stuff we've totally spaced!

This brings me to the other lesson I got from the tragedy of the plaster Buddha. The journey from misery to Peace isn't an easy, gradual journey. From where we're standing, we can't just stroll into Heaven. As we bought into the delusions of the Misery Conspiracy, we have built brick-by-brick and loveless-thought-by-loveless-thought a wall of insecurities, resentments and jealousies, self that we have completely lost sight of our deeper nature. Even if someone tells us the truth, we scoff at them as full of crap. *Take responsibility for my emotions? I can't! How can I be happy when they're making me angry!*

Unfortunately, it often takes a tragedy to get us to see past the illusion of our bodies and our personalities. For some of us, it takes hitting bottom with alcoholism. Other people bust through the plaster with a serious illness or the loss of a loved one. It may even take a series of disasters before we're ready to take a look at what's underneath the veneer of our little selves.

If you have lost custody of your kids or your Uncle Charlie loved you just a little too much or your anorexia gets you mistaken for a P.O.W., it's time to take your worldview and ever-so-gently smash the Hell out of it! In order to get back in touch with the One Self, to experience the Kingdom of Heaven within us, our world of illusions has to be smashed and shattered beyond repair. It's only when we have no more illusions to hide behind that we take a peek at what's underneath. That's when the miracle happens. That's when we find that Peace that passes all understanding.

Chapter 46:
Stressing About the Holidays

Too often we rob ourselves of Peace in the very experiences designed to bring us closer to Peace. The insanity of the Misery Conspiracy takes something holy like the holidays at the end of the year and turns them into a full-contact ragefest.

The end of the year is a bizarre time, driving many of us to do what we would not otherwise do. We buy too much. We eat too much. A lot of us drink too much. I hear people say that they love the holidays, but then they go on a rant about how stressed out they are about it. Shopping. Travel plans. Fruit cakes. Dysfunctional families. Yada yada yada...

Okay, people. Pay very close attention now. If the holidays stress you out, YOU'RE MISSING THE WHOLE POINT!!!!! If you're more focused on finding that perfect gift for your mother than you are on letting go of your judgments of her, then the purpose of the holidays, including Thanksgiving, Hanukkah, Christmas, Solstice and Kwanzaa is totally lost on you.

The holidays are an opportunity to refocus our minds on gratitude, miracles, faith, meditation, prayer, hope, values and renewal. It's a chance to take a personal inventory of where you are doing well emotionally and spiritually and where you still need a lot of work.

My personal term for the winter holidays is the Season of Light. Many spiritual traditions use the symbol of light for this time of year. Many cultures light candles as part of their seasonal celebration. The Light represents the Divine within us; pure and without form.

I was raised in a typical Christian home, where Christmas meant fighting the crowds at the mall to buy presents you couldn't afford, often for people we didn't really care about. Yes, there were some traditions that I still cherish, such as my mother's home-made treats and watching *A Charlie Brown Christmas* for the hundredth time. But the focus was always the presents and always left me wanting for something more meaningful; something that didn't require exchanging gifts or buying batteries.

It took me a long time to muster the courage not to do the whole gift-buying, gift-giving rat race, and instead focus on the spiritual aspects on the Season of Light. I was afraid that people would think I was being selfish or contrary. However, the response I get during the holidays when I explain that I don't exchange gifts is one of envy. People say they wish they could do the same.

I make a practice of giving unexpected gifts to people throughout the year, with no expectation of reciprocation. To me, it makes the giving that I do more heartfelt and more genuine. If a friend or even a stranger needs money, I have it to spare, I give it with no strings attached. I volunteer my time for different organizations and programs. That's just me. And I have found that when I need it, people have been there for me, as well.

If the holiday shopping sprees get you down, then quit playing that game. If you just aren't up for cooking an elaborate holiday dinner for your entire extended family, then don't! Find a restaurant that will be open or have T.V. dinners. Use the time for sharing and loving rather than shopping or any other tradition that doesn't have any spiritual merit. Take this season off to celebrate the Season of Light in whatever tradition really speaks to your Spirit.

Chapter 47:
Transforming Our Childhoods

One of the remarkable qualities of Divine Peace is its ability to shape not only the present and the future, but also to change the past. Okay, you can't exactly change the past. That car you totaled three years ago when you hit an icy patch and had a close encounter with a stop sign isn't going to magically reappear in your driveway. However, you can dramatically change the negative impact in your life and even use it to increase your Peace of Mind.

I've seen a bumper sticker (and you've probably seen it, too) that reads, "It's never too late to have a Happy childhood." I'm finding that this is truer than I realized. And the teddy bear that I have slept with every night for the past decade will testify to that.

Many of us had difficult, even traumatic, childhoods. Maybe you were physically, sexually, or emotionally abused. Maybe you feel you were neglected by your parents. Maybe you found yourself lost in the foster care system. But however painful it was when you were young, you have the power in this moment to transform it.

We can't necessarily go back in time and stop the "bad things" from happening. On the other hand, we *can* change the purpose they served. We can use the crap from our younger days as fertilizer for growing our more Peaceful, enlightened selves. And some of us have a *lot* of fertilizer to spread.

When I was in ninth grade, I had a girlfriend. I honestly can't remember her name, but I will call her "Stacy". We were both into drama and acting in school plays. We read abstract (and utterly incomprehensible) poetry to each other. We went to see independent films with subtitles and depressing endings. After about a month and a half, she took me to my first showing of *Rocky Horror Picture Show*. Oh my God!

If you've never seen *Rocky Horror*, I won't spoil the experience. I will say that as a 13-year old kid, I wasn't expecting the bizarreness that has made the film the cult classic that it is. But as if the movie wasn't shocking enough, Stacy picked this time to dump me.

Right in the middle of the film, she changed seats and started cozying up to some guy from our class, who happened to be in the theatre at the time. I almost threw up right there. How could you bring a date to a flick like *Rocky Horror* and then dump her in the middle of it? No warning. Just, *boom*! Dumped! That has to be against the official dumping rules.

I was devastated. For two months I hardly left my room. I just listed to the soundtrack to the movie *Fame* over and over, crying and pining for Stacy the heartbreaker. To this day, the song "Is It Okay" brings a tear to my eyes. But I got over it.

I realize that getting dumped isn't the worst thing that can happen to a kid. Too many children these days are abused, neglected or suffer from devastating illnesses or injuries. But regardless of the severity of the traumas we experienced as kids, we have the power to change the effects they have had on our lives.

We can use the traumas, including the really awful ones, as lessons in letting go of anger and hurt. We can see our perpetrators as teachers whose purpose was to show us where we've blocked Love. Through their own callous, sometimes brutal behavior, they can teach us about the deeper power of Forgiveness. And this has the effect of undoing all of the damage we thought we suffered as children.

When we consciously make the effort to transform the past, to redefine what it means to us, we free ourselves from the grip of the Misery Conspiracy. We can rip that "victim" label and even the "survivor" label off our chest, and instead identify as the Divine Beings we are. The next time someone brings up a past hurt, we will no longer be thrown into that same emotional Hell that has haunted us into our adult lives.

Getting dumped by Stacy wasn't a bad thing, even though it hurt a lot. It forced me to look at myself. It taught me some things about dating. It taught me that my identity isn't tied up with who I'm with. It taught me that even when my world seems to come crashing down, when the people and things that I'm emotionally attached to are ripped away, I get past it. The wounds will heal, and I will be okay.

If you were abused as a child, you can use it as an excuse not to trust anyone (not recommended) or as a way to learn how to trust your intuition. I'm amazed at how intuitive and perceptive survivors of abuse are (including myself), and how reluctant we are to trust that intuition. It's time to turn those traumas around and use them to our advantage.

It's never too late to have a Happy childhood. Trust me on this. When I separated from my ex-husband, I bought me a teddy bear. It helped to have something to hold in that empty bed. And not only do I still have that bear, but Eileen has one too.

I still keep a box of crayons and coloring books handy. It can be really helpful when I get stuck creatively or just need to vent some anger. Like I said, sometimes Barbie needs a blue face!

Your happy childhood is waiting for you. Wanna play?

Chapter 48:
The Illusion of Anger

As a kid, I was always the shortest kid in my class. Not only was I short for my age, but most people in my class were nearly a year older than me because of where my birthday falls. And because young kids are always such angels, my diminutive stature frequently made me a magnet for bullies. I think my mother still has my collection of "Kick Me" signs that were taped to my back.

My most frequent nemesis was Brian Hensley. From the day he moved in across the street, Brian was gunning for me. I tried being friends with him, but he seemed pre-programmed for aggression. My mother's advice of "Just ignore him" wasn't exactly helpful. The guy was a bully with my name at the top of his hit list. Kind of hard to ignore something like that.

But my mom did tell me something that, while not terribly helpful at the time, has provided some insight into situations later in life. She said, "You have to understand, he's had a hard life." And he had. He suffered from childhood diabetes and his father reminded me of a rabid bulldog with a personality disorder. I suppose that can have an adverse effect on a child's disposition.

Mind you, this little insight didn't help me fend off bullies, particularly Brian Hensley. But years later, it helped me understand that there was something underneath, spurring on the angry, violent behavior. As adults, we tend to forget this because all we see is the hate and venom. Consequently, angry, violent people are very hard for most of us to Love and Forgive.

Remember the time you saw a woman sitting somewhere crying by herself. What was your natural impulse? You wanted to go over there and ask what's wrong, right? You felt compelled to offer assistance, and if you did, kudos to you! But would your response have been the same if instead of crying, she was visibly angry, cursing to herself, or pounding the table?

When hurt is turned outward in the form of anger and violence, Compassion is often the last thing on our mind. We see the angry person as a threat, as part of the problems in the world, whether they are juvenile delinquents, ruthless killers, or just an angry woman mumbling curses under her breathe. We have no Love to give them because we feel they don't deserve it.

If someone acts like a wounded, cowering puppy, our hearts go out to him. But if he is snarling, snapping and foaming at the mouth, we are more apt to respond with apathy and disdain. And this is understandable! But if we don't want people snarling at us, we have to do more than call snarl back.

Anger is confusing because it looks defiant, strong, unafraid and powerful. We can't see the hurt because we associate hurt with weakness, fear and surrender. We forget that the reason people are angry is because they *are* hurting. The reality is 180° away from the mask they are showing the world. Angry people drive people away because they are afraid of being hurt worse.

The enlightened response to anger is Compassion, Patience and Forgiveness. The goal is to reach the angry person and help them work through their anger if possible. Diffuse the bomb rather than simply running away from it. This isn't always easy, or even possible, especially if our encounter with such a person is brief. But just the simple act of acknowledging their feelings of anger, just saying "I hear you", can be enough to at least tip the balance in the other direction.

There wasn't a lot I could do for Brian Hensley as a kid. I was just trying not to get beat up. But as an adult, there is a lot I can do for the Brian Hensley look-alikes that I encounter in my daily life. I can listen to their rants, appreciate their pain, imagine their difficult history, and respond with understanding. I can't fix them, but I can remind them that they are worth loving, and that there is a better way to deal with a dysfunctional past.

Don't let the illusion of anger blind you to someone's pain. Keep yourself safe from violence, but let your heart be open to Forgiving. Remind yourself that this is a person who has been traumatized, and who is in desperate need for Love.

Chapter 49:
Stumbling Through Wisdom

The road to Peace is not a straight line. It more closely resembles the artistic stylings of a 2-year old with a box of crayons. It isn't neat. It doesn't stay within the lines that we think it should. It's chaotic and wild, with scribbles going everywhere. And sometimes Barbie ends up with a blue face and green arms and purple feet.

Part of the reason that our spiritual journeys to the wonderful land of Bliss are so erratic is that Divine Truth is so far beyond our current understanding. So much of it doesn't translate into our Misery Conspiracy-oriented worldview. This explains why the few enlightened teachers over the centuries (e.g. Jesus, Buddha, Rumi, etc.) have often left us scratching our heads incomprehensibly, and occasionally frustrating us to the point of wanting to nail them to a tree.

When it comes to religion, I've always been a bit of a nomad. This is hardly surprising considering that my mother's family is Jewish and my father's is Irish Catholic. And when we left the Catholic Church in favor of the Episcopal Church (I was ten at the time), my religious journey began in earnest. Since then, I have been Baptist, Pagan, Buddhist, and a member of various other organizations, including Church of Christ, Metropolitan Community Church, Unity and the 12-Step recovery programs.

About a year before I got sober, I discovered *A Course in Miracles*. After reading Marianne Williamson's fabulously transformative *A Return to Love* (my "gateway drug" to the Course), I attempted to plumb the depths of this radical spiritual teaching. At the time, I was struggling with alcoholism, my sexuality, and my dysfunctional marriage. I was desperate to find a way to stop the immense pain I had been feeling for much of my life.

When I first started reading the Course, I had a difficult time understanding it. It used familiar terms like "miracle," "ego," and "forgiveness" in very unfamiliar ways. So for years I would pick it up, read about 30 pages and then put it down again in frustration. I just couldn't grasp the concepts. I was drawn to its wisdom but could not seem to find the key to unlock it.

It wasn't until I had five years of sobriety under my belt that I managed to unlock some of its secrets. I trudged through the Text (the first major section) and stepped through the 365 daily lessons of the Workbook (the second section). I finally emerged on the far side of the Manual for Teachers (the final section). This process took me nearly two years of dedicated study.

I didn't always understand what I was reading, and some concepts still are beyond my level of comprehension. But in the end, I discovered how to let go of my fears and judgments, to change my perspectives, and ultimately to find a deeper Peace of Mind.

But understanding the theory is, as I've said, only part of the battle. Whatever our form of religious expression maybe, we have to apply the spiritual principles to our life situation for them to help. And we have to apply them a lot! And as I said before this process is chaotic and involves repeating the same lessons over and over until learned.

I have actively worked on overcoming the issues that sent me into an emotional funk for much of my life. In this effort I have made a lot of progress. And yet every once in a great while, a situation will really throw me. When this happens, my mind goes back into "victim" mode. My mind dredges up a trauma from my past (and there are so many to choose from), flooding me with overwhelming fear, hopelessness, and despair.

I know what to do to take care of myself, when this happens. Call someone. Pray. Meditate. Read something positive and inspirational. Go to a 12-step meeting. That's what my Hurricane and Doldrums lists are for. Most of the time, I use these tools and get re-centered. But not always.

There are still times (thankfully rare now) when my thought process is so wrought with fear that I have no desire to take care of myself. I am drawn to the familiarity of my old insane thought process, like a long awaited reunion with the kid that taught you how to smoke or gave you your first sip of Mad Dog 20/20. Yick!

In those times, I don't want to do the responsible thing. I just want to crawl into a hole and disappear, and at the same time show the people around me how much they have hurt me. I want to sulk. I turn the Victim-ometer up all the way.

It is difficult when I'm in this state to find the motivation to take care of myself, to bridge the gap between fear and Love. When my ego mind is running the show, the desire to reach out for help seems nonexistent, or at least pushed so far back in my mind as to be inaccessible. I know that if I pray and meditate, the pain and despair will vanish like the morning mist. Yet doing so would require that I give up my self-pity, which my ego loves to wallow in.

Fortunately, these pity parties are rare and brief. I am blessed to have friends who call me on my stinkin'-thinkin'. And they have no hesitation about using my own words and teachings against me. They will say, "If it was me having this problem, what would you tell me to do?" or "Didn't you tell me last week that what people think about you is none of your business? Then why are you upset over this lousy review from the New York Times?" I hate it when they do that, but they're right. And I get over it.

To prevent yourself from falling back into the old "poor me" routines and pulling out the old "worthless" tapes from your dysfunctional childhood (and we all had dysfunctional child-hoods), use the tools in your spiritual toolbox regularly. Use them so often that they become deeply ingrained in my mind. Make the grooves so deep in your consciousness that they show up as dimples and laugh lines on your face.

I've been to so many recovery meetings that the protocols of the meetings show up unexpectedly in other situations. When I attend non-recovery meetings and someone introduces herself with something like "Hi, my name is Delores," I automatically respond, "Hi Delores", as if I'm at an AA meeting. And then I notice everyone looking at me as if I have rabid monkeys on my head.

I have a meditation track with a gong at the beginning and end that I ripped from one of my CDs and have put on my MP3 player. I have listened to it so many times, that anytime I hear a gong on the T.V. or radio, I feel this urge to focus on my breathing.

And I have practiced some mantras so many times that I frequently catch myself singing in Sanskrit as I'm driving down the road. When Eileen catches me doing it, she laughs. And when I claim to be humming the Battlestar Galactica theme, she says, "Yeah, right!" She knows me too well.

This is the real meaning of "spiritual practice". By making your spiritual tools a regular part of your daily routine, these emotional spirals occur less often and when they do occur, they don't last as long. You just naturally take the necessary steps to return to a more loving state of mind.

The late poet/artist Portia Nelson illustrated this process in her poem, "Autobiography in Five Short Chapters," which was published in her book, *There's a Hole in My Sidewalk*. In this poem, she described how, when we face a major issue like depression, addiction, etc., we are angry and in denial and have no tools with which to help ourselves get out of our "hole."

However, as we work on understanding the underlying dynamics and learn how to utilize spiritual tools, our time "in the hole" becomes dramatically shorter. Through continued use of these tools, we no longer fall in the hole and our path changes so that there are no longer any holes to fall into.

This is the road to Peace. It's not a straight road, but there are a few straight-aways. There are also lots of twists and turns and hills and potholes. But these road hazards have always been there. As we learn to recognize the traps of the Misery Conspiracy, as we learn the life lessons that we have been missing, as we use the tools in our spiritual toolbox with greater and greater dexterity, we will navigate around the road hazards. And eventually, the hazards will no longer show up. All we will experience is Peace.

Conclusion:
Subversive Love

Well, you've done it. You've reached the last chapter of the book. Well done! Are you enlightened yet? Do you glow with wisdom? Does gravity lose its grip on you as you meditate? Do crowds of homeless people and lepers follow you everywhere, hanging on your every word? Okay, not yet. But you must admit, you feel a little bit better. You're smiling more. And that outfit looks fantastic on you! Where did you get it?

Even though you haven't yet mastered walking on water (I believe it's offered next semester, if you're interested), you have certainly learned that you have a right to be Happy. You don't have to wait for anything outside of you to change. You can experience Joy and Peace right now.

And now you want to tell the world, don't you? You want to expose everyone to the truth about the Misery Conspiracy. You have become a proud member of the Spiritual Underground. Your "Heretic" pin has been ordered and should arrive in 5-10 business days (just kidding!).

Realize that unless you're some spiritual savant, you will have lots of practice to endure before you reach enlightened status. And not everyone will immediately be charmed by your newfound understanding of spiritual dynamics. It's amazing how fervently and sometimes violently people will defend their right to be miserable. My advice is to let them stay there as long as they want. If they want to wallow in the mud, let them. It's good for their skin. But leave the gate open for them for when they get tired of it and want to leave.

The Buddha Shakyamuni (the skinny Peaceful Buddha, not the fat, jolly Buddha) did not start out as a spiritual leader. That came much later. Long before he became an enlightened master, he was a prince in India.

He was raised in a sheltered environment, far away from the ravages of sickness, poverty and death. He did not even know such miserable conditions existed. It was not until he insisted (against his father's wishes) to be allowed to see the people that they governed, that he ventured outside the castle walls.

When he saw the suffering of the people in his kingdom, it broke his heart. He gave up the luxuries of a royal life and ran off to find a way to end the suffering of humanity. His family thought he was crazy to chase such a dream. Why give up a life of opulence to going chasing after the impossible? But such is the subversive nature of Love.

Jesus of Nazareth, too, was subversive in his ministry. He blatantly defied the legalistic and often loveless power structure of the fundamentalist priesthood. He healed people on the Sabbath. He forgave people their sins. He taught the importance of respecting non-Jews, including Samaritans and Romans. His message of Love was considered a threat by those in power. It exposed the corruption and hypocrisy of those in the service of the Misery Conspiracy.

And now you, too, realize that the Misery Conspiracy is full of crap (good thing you dusted off the Anti-Misery Conspiracy Crap Detector, otherwise known as your intuition). You no longer want to be miserable. You no longer want to play the Conspiracy's stupid mind games. The pain of staying the same has overcome our fear of change. You've reach the turning point. You have glimpsed the One Self. This is the place where we demand radical change and are willing to consider new possibilities.

Now you reconsider the alternative to loveless thinking. You let go of guilt, judgments, fear, and self-pity. You admit your shortcomings, make amends to those you have harmed and seek for a power greater than the worn-out, limited image of your little self.

You honor your boundaries and let go of trying to control others. You see yourself and the world in a whole new way, as part of the One Self. You have become united with the Consciousness of Unconditional Love.

When you open yourself to Love, these are some of the Truths you will realize:

- You are good enough, smart enough, thin enough, beautiful enough, rich enough, and holy enough.
- You are not your body, your job, your religion or your possessions.
- In order for you to gain, no one has to lose. And if you can help someone else in the process, you will gain that much more.
- You are Divine. You are part of the One Self.
- You are not guilty (that speeding ticket not withstanding).
- The One Self wants you to let go of your fears and be in unity with your Divine Nature.
- The Consciousness of Unconditional Love Loves women, people of color (including those of us that are rosy beige with brown polka dots), atheists, agnostics, pagans, and gay people just as much as He loves other people. We are all part of the One Self.
- The One Self is beyond gender.
- The One Self is more concerned with your openness to Love and Peace than any behaviors.
- The One Self has no ego, and could never be offended by our mistakes or defiance.
- The One Self Loves you in spite of your mistakes, because It knows you are not your mistakes.
- The One Self knows that Hell is simply our self-created separation from the Divine within us.
- If you don't learn everything about Love in this life, then you can do it in the next one or the one after that. Eventu-

ally you will embody the One Self. An eternity in Hell is not an option.

- The One Self would never punish you. You do enough of that to yourself.
- The One Self has designed the Universe to support our continued growth to Bliss. It allows for war, disease, and the illusion of death only to teach us that they are unnecessary.
- There are infinite ways to God/Heaven/Enlightenment.
- No one has a monopoly on Truth. Use wisdom wherever you find it; in the Bible, in a movie or written on a bathroom stall.
- Anger, judgment and/or violence in the name of God are clear evidence of a lack of understanding.
- Men and women are equally holy because gender is simply a temporary form.
- No end ever justifies withholding love or acting out of fear.
- Might does not always equal right.
- Violence can get you what you want...if what you want is to be miserable.
- Nothing outside of you can make you Happy.
- Judgment, unforgiveness, resentments, and worry produce nothing but upset.
- Fear accomplishes no good thing.
- Love is the most powerful force in the universe.
- There are no legitimate reasons not to Love someone.
- You never need a reason to be Happy. Happiness is always your right to claim anytime you want.
- You can be just as Happy at 8:00 AM on a Monday as you can at 5:00 PM on Friday.
- Work is an opportunity to learn how to Love more.
- Success or the accumulation of wealth is a sign of nothing. How you use them is very telling, however.
- You can influence what other people do or think, but you never have control of anything but your actions and your attitudes.

It would be tempting to tell you that when you start living this new way of Love and Compassion that life instantly becomes a "happily ever after" story. It doesn't. As our perception of our world changes, we become aware of habits that need to end (like drinking and manipulating people), places that only serve our addictions (like bars), and people that don't respect us and/or trigger our hot buttons. We find that we have to set boundaries with some people, and they don't often respond well when we do. When you begin to make such radical changes, resistance is inevitable. This is the epitome of the Misery Conspiracy

Once when my ex-husband and I were separated, he asked to come over to my apartment to talk. In the hopes of healing our relationship, I agreed. What can I say? I was having one of those "You had me at 'Hello'" moments.

We discussed things in an unemotional, non-blaming way for about 15 minutes. Then he started into his old shaming routine. I had enough sobriety time under my belt that I realized that I needed to set a boundary. I told him he needed to leave.

Somehow I managed to get him out of the apartment, but a few minutes later, he started pounding on the outside of the door. He demanded to be let back in. I refused. I called my friend Terri instead. I needed backup if I was going to maintain this boundary. Terri had always been there for me, and she talked to me while Ray was doing his Big, Bad Wolf imitation.

For twenty minutes, he continued to pound and plead, but I maintained my boundary, thanks to Terri. I didn't play the game. I didn't even respond to his rants. I just ignored him and talk to Terri until he went away.

It's odd. Crazy, emotionally unhealthy people don't like it when you get healthy. And they really resent you call them on passive-aggressive behavior. Not that it's your job to work their recovery, but if they ask why you stopped playing their sick games, tell them (diplomatically if possible).

When you stand up for love and compassion, this world will not always reflect the same back to you because it hasn't yet learned what you have. Just be patient while applying the principles you have learned. Take care of yourself and trust the process.

I saw a poster at a 12-step meeting that describes the stages that people often go through after they've become sober or changed their lives in a similarly profound way. It said, "First things get better. Then they get worse. Then they get different. Then they get real. Then they get real different."

That really captures the continuous, yet ever-changing process of living beyond the insanity of the Misery Conspiracy. We go through good times and tough times, and exciting times, and profound times. It's all part of the Universal Process of Healing. It's as true for you as it is for me.

The Misery Conspiracy will throw everything it has at us; guilt, lies, violence, despair and the occasional bad review. When we overcome our insanity, people sometimes resent us because our Peace shows them how insane *they* are. They wonder why you should be so flippin' Happy, when they are miserable. Rather than look within and take responsibility for their own crazed thinking, they would rather bring you down. That's what makes Love seem so subversive. It threatens to expose people to change. It reminds them of their need to take responsibility for their own thoughts. To many, that's frightening.

Hang in there, though. When people respond with anger, fear, distrust, rage, and even violence, it is only because they are still stuck in the Conspiracy's thinking. They still perceive the world, and specifically you, as a threat. No one has taught them that it's all a lie. No one has loved them enough to help them break through the illusions. What would happen if you made the decision to Love them regardless of their insanity?

The good news is that as we become more aware of the spiritual dynamics in our lives (the effects of judgment, the power of Forgiveness, etc.) and begin to use the tools available to us (prayer, meditation, letting go of control, etc.), the twists and turns in life have less of an effect on our Peace of Mind. We lose the manic-depressive mood swings that the Misery Conspiracy brings to our lives. We become much more stable than we were when we thought our Happiness depended on our circumstances.

For reasons not yet apparent, you are exactly where you need to be. No, you're not being punished. There are simply lessons to be learned and right here is the best place for you to learn them. The Universe is designed to support your belief system. You can use it to further your belief in fear and separation or in Love and unity. It's your choice. And whatever you choose is what you will get.

Well, that's it. I've no more lessons to teach you. At least not until my next book. Until then, take these lessons and practice them...a lot. That's why it's called having a spiritual practice, remember? Perfection comes a bit later in the program. Until we meet again, trust the process.

Peas and hominy,
Dharmashanti

About the Author

Dharmashanti has been a spiritual teacher for many years and has authored several articles on spiritual dynamics. Having overcome alcoholism, codependency and depression, she had dedicated her life to helping others do the same.

Dharmashanti has intensely studied the wisdom of several spiritual traditions, including Buddhism, *A Course in Miracles*, and the teachings of Alcoholics Anonymous. She actively participates in online spiritual discussion groups and in women's spiritual circles in Phoenix, Arizona, where she resides.

Through her writing, speaking and other creative ventures, she teaches people how reconnect to our Spiritual Source and achieve a profound inner Peace and Joy. She frequently combines spiritual wisdom with her quirky sense of humor as a way of connecting with people that is both inspiring and down-to-earth.

If you liked *Fight the Misery Conspiracy*, be sure to check out her website at www.dharmashanti.com. Read articles she's written. Share your thoughts on her blog (online journal). And shop the boutique for T-shirts, bumper stickers and more with positive messages. Join the Spiritual Underground! Fight the Misery Conspiracy! Reclaim your Happiness.